Pregnancy & Childbirth

The Basic Illustrated Guide

Pregnancy & Childbirth

The Basic Illustrated Guide

Margaret Martin, M.P.H.

Founder, Pregnancy and Natural Childbirth Education Center

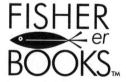

FISHER
BOOKS™

Publishers: Bill Fisher
Howard W. Fisher
Helen Fisher

Managing Editor: Sarah Trotta

Cover design: FifthStreet*design*
Cover photo: ©TMS/Jose Pelaez
Production: Deanie Wood
Randy Schultz

Published by Fisher Books
4239 W. Ina Road, Suite 101
Tucson, Arizona 85741
(520) 744-6110

First published in 1991 as *The Illustrated Book of Pregnancy and Childbirth*. Text and illustrations copyright ©1991, ©1997 by Margaret Martin

Printed in U.S.A.
Printing 10 9 8 7 6 5 4 3 2 1

Library of Congress Cataloging-in Publication Data
Martin, Margaret, 1954-
    Pregnancy and childbirth: the basic illustrated guide / Margaret Martin.
        p. cm.
Previously published with title: The illustrated book of pregnancy and childbirth.
    Includes index.
    ISBN 1-55561-114-1
1. Childbirth. 2. Pregnancy. I. Martin, Margaret, 1954-
Illustrated book of pregnancy and childbirth. II. Title.
    RG525.M3338 1997
    618.2--DC21   96-37277
                                    CIP

Fisher Books are available at special discounts when purchased in bulk quantities for businesses, associations, institutions or sales promotions. Please call our Special Sales Department at 800-255-1514.

Notice: The information in this book is true and complete to the best of our knowledge. It is offered with no guarantees on the part of the author or Fisher Books. Author and publisher disclaim all liability in connection with use of this book.

FOR ALL
OUR FAMILIES

CONTENTS

FOREWORD

I have been teaching childbirth classes for many years. But each new group I meet surprises me by knowing so little about the workings of their bodies, about childbirth, about labor and delivery. There is certainly ample information available in books and magazine articles. And most people have been told in high school or college about the extraordinary engineering feat our bodies perform when we give birth to a child. But in spite of all the information, old wives' tales and misconceptions are passed on from generation to generation, from woman to woman.

Margaret Martin's book fills in the gaps in so many people's knowledge. Her book describes in simple language and with wonderfully clear illustrations what is happening in our bodies when we are expecting a baby. The author tells what to look for in the various stages and phases of labor and delivery, and then continues to discuss the first week after birth.

She includes a chapter on nutrition, and though many of us know what is meant by "healthy eating," few of us know much about healthy eating once we are pregnant.

Pregnancy and childbirth are considered to be among the peak experiences in a person's life. Both physically and emotionally we need a guide to see us through and help us understand what changes, both physical and emotional, are likely to occur.

This book is such a guide for every woman who is expecting a child.

ELISABETH BING, FACCE

ACKNOWLEDGMENTS

I am deeply grateful to the many hundreds of pregnant women and their families whom I have educated throughout the years, for allowing me to share in their journey through pregnancy and childbirth. This journey, more often than not, brings out the best that men and women have to offer—love, hope, determination, patience, faith and a generous optimism regarding the future. Sharing in this journey has been an incomparably rewarding adventure.

I must also acknowledge the pioneers of modern birth education, Dr. Grantley Dick Read of England, whose work in the early part of this century was followed by Dr. Fernand Lamaze, in France, and Dr. Robert Bradley, in the United States; Elisabeth Bing, whose vision and tireless efforts are responsible for the training of Lamaze educators throughout the United States through A.S.P.O. (American Society for Psychoprophylaxis in Obstetrics), and Marjie and Jay Hathaway, who, with Dr. Bradley, have worked to train Bradley educators throughout the United States through the A.A.H.C.C. (American Academy of Husband-Coached Childbirth), and who initially trained me.

I warmly thank my husband, my children and my parents for their patience and loving support.

I affectionately acknowledge Emilie Sparks, Sylvia Solana, Christine Vega, M.P.H., R.D., and Tomi Mikkelsen, whose commitment, friendship and work helped me bring the Pregnancy and Natural Childbirth Education Center to life in Los Angeles in the late 1970s and early '80s, and Drs. Stephen Brunton, John George, Uziel Reiss, N.B. Ettinghausen and the other doctors, nurses and educators who formed the core of the Center's Advisory Board.

I thank Laura Blanchette for her invaluable technical assistance in preparing the copy for this book and for her patience and unflagging good spirits.

Thanks are due, too, for ongoing inspiration provided by the wonderful staff and students of U.C.L.A.'s School of Public Health, whose dedicated enthusiasm and committed work daily improve both the health and quality of life of individuals and families throughout the U.S. and around the world.

And special thanks to my friend and mentor, the late Norman Cousins, whose kind interest helped to make the publication of this book a reality.

INTRODUCTION

Education provides options. It makes choices possible. Education adds color and dimension to a black-and-white, two-dimensional view of the world.

Some women have asked me, "Why learn about pregnancy, labor and birth? It's all just going to happen by itself, anyway!"

And these women are right! Something's going to happen "anyway," that's for sure! The question is what?

The following complaints of pregnancy can be prevented entirely, or drastically reduced:

- headaches
- nausea
- heartburn
- indigestion
- constipation
- backache

and a host of others. This is only one reason to learn about pregnancy.

When you learn about pregnancy and good prenatal care (including excellent nutrition and exercise) you can help keep your baby from coming too soon and from being too small. You can do a lot to reduce or eliminate serious risks for the child.

Low birth weight (babies born under 5-1/2 pounds) is associated with a large increase in birth defects. Low birth weight can often be prevented.

You can also learn to eliminate many other risks, which otherwise could lead to a longer, more difficult labor, birth and recovery.

Giving birth without knowing what's going on is kind of like going on a roller-coaster ride with a bag over your head. Sure, you get to the end of the ride, all right. But flinging along, without knowing what to expect, can be a frightening, even horrifying experience.

It's important to realize that the emotions of a woman in labor play a very large part in the progress of that labor. Labor is controlled by hormones released within a woman's body. The release of these hormones is determined to a very large degree by the emotional condition of the laboring woman. If she is frightened and tense, her body can actually work against itself. Labor can slow down. Contractions (of the uterus) can become less effective.

If she is relaxed and in good spirits, her labor can progress more rapidly and easily.

For this reason alone, many doctors today vigorously recommend that women attend classes about pregnancy and birth. They observe an enormous difference in the progress of the labors of educated, relaxed women.

We can be frightened of things we do not understand. Once we understand them, we can manage them and even enjoy them.

For many women, pregnancy can also be a lonely time. She is always aware of being pregnant. She cannot move, think or breathe without that awareness. But it's not so for everyone else. This illustrated book makes it easy for every member of the family to understand what's going on in pregnancy, labor and birth. This helps the entire family to provide much-needed support and encouragement to the pregnant woman and a better welcome for the child.

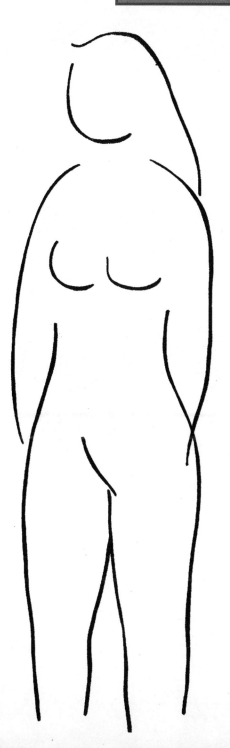

To understand how pregnancy and birth happen, it is necessary to understand a little about a woman's body.

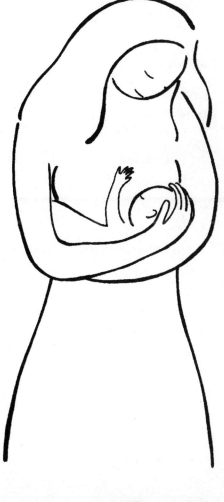

Body Openings

(1) The **urethra** is the passage leading from the bladder, through which urine flows out of the body.

(2) The **vagina** is the passage leading to the uterus. The **vagina** is also called the **birth canal**. This is because a baby must pass from the uterus, through the vagina, to come out into the world.

(3) The **rectum** is the lowest part of the large intestine. Solid body wastes (bowel movements) pass through this passage and out of the body.

(4) The **bladder** is the little triangle-shaped bag that holds urine, the body's liquid waste.

(5) The **uterus (womb)** is the muscle-bag in which a baby grows. It is shown here before pregnancy, when it is about the size of a small pear.

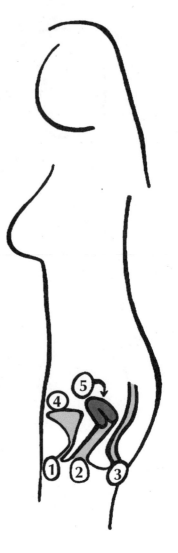

Bones

(6) The **pubic bone** in the lower front part of the body protects the *bladder* behind it.

(7) The **spine** or **backbone**.

(8) The **tail bone** is the lowest part of the spine. It is also called the **coccyx.**

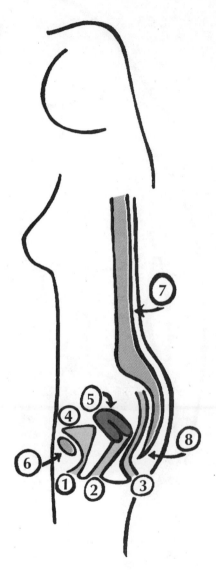

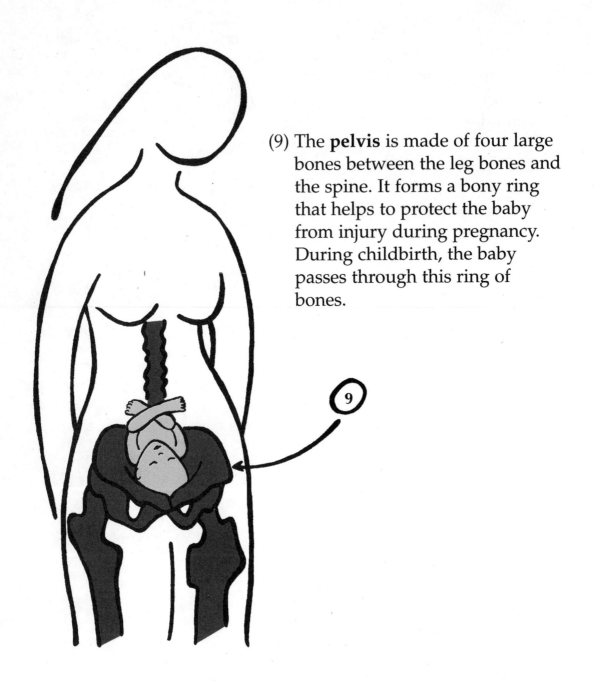

(9) The **pelvis** is made of four large bones between the leg bones and the spine. It forms a bony ring that helps to protect the baby from injury during pregnancy. During childbirth, the baby passes through this ring of bones.

Menstruation

The Monthly "Period"

When a girl becomes a young woman, her body prepares itself for the possibility of one day becoming a mother.

Part of this preparation is the growth of her breasts. Other signs are the appearance of hair under her arms and in the pubic area, and the appearance of **menstruation**.

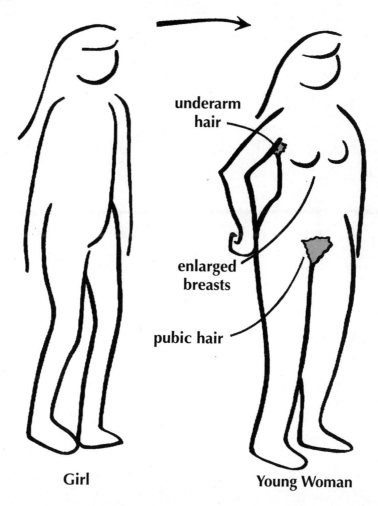

underarm hair

enlarged breasts

pubic hair

Girl

Young Woman

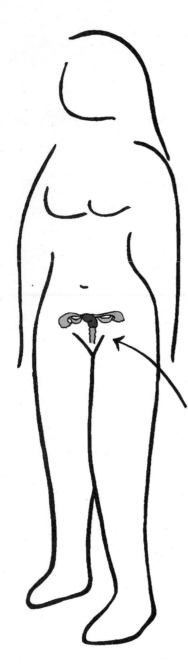

A woman carries eggs **(ova)** in two little sacs inside her body called **ovaries**. When she is born she already has all the eggs she ever will have.

One **ovary** is on either side of the **uterus** (womb). Each ovary is connected to the uterus by a thin **tube**. (**Fallopian tubes**—named after Gabriel Fallopius, who first described them.)

Ovulation

Each month one egg ripens and bursts from one of the ovaries into the Fallopian tube. The ovaries take turns. Each one sends out one ripe egg every other month.

Ovulation is the time a ripe egg leaves the ovary. It occurs only once each month, usually about 14 days after the first day of the last **period**.

The **menstrual period** occurs every 24 to 32 days, and lasts about three to six days. Most women have 28-day menstrual cycles. (Their menstrual periods start every 28 days.)

menstrual period

cycle	
28-day	1 2 3 4 5 6 7 8 9 10 11 12 13 **14** 15 16 17 18 19 20 21 22 23 24 25 26 27 28
26-day	1 2 3 4 5 6 7 8 9 10 11 12 13 **14** 15 16 17 18 19 20 21 22 23 24 25 26
30-day	1 2 3 4 5 6 7 8 9 10 11 12 13 **14** 15 16 17 18 19 20 21 22 23 24 25 26 27 28 29 30

Ovulation usually occurs
close to this date.

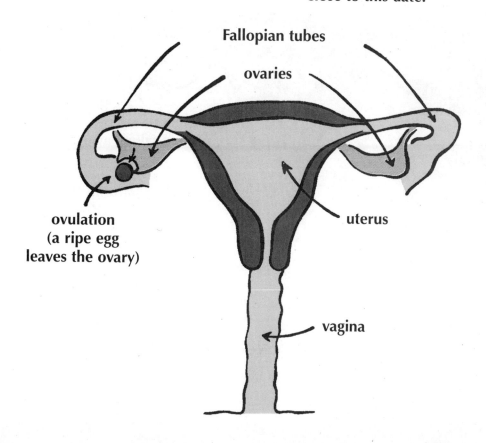

Fallopian tubes

ovaries

**ovulation
(a ripe egg
leaves the ovary)**

uterus

vagina

The uterus prepares itself for the coming egg by building up layers of blood to nourish the egg.

If the egg is *not* fertilized (does not meet up with a live sperm within about 24 hours after it leaves the ovary) the egg will fall apart and the blood built up inside the uterus will fall away—out of the uterus, through the vagina, and out of the woman's body.

This monthly loss of the unfertilized egg and blood is called **menstruation**, or more commonly, a woman's monthly **period.** It occurs about 400 times in a woman's life, beginning in her early teens, and ending sometime 30 to 40 years later.

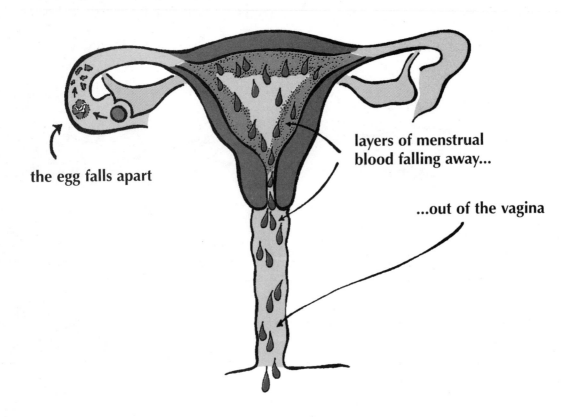

the egg falls apart

layers of menstrual blood falling away...

...out of the vagina

Conception

When sperm are deposited in or near the opening of the
vagina and one of them meets a ripe egg in the Fallopian tube,
conception occurs. The egg becomes fertilized.

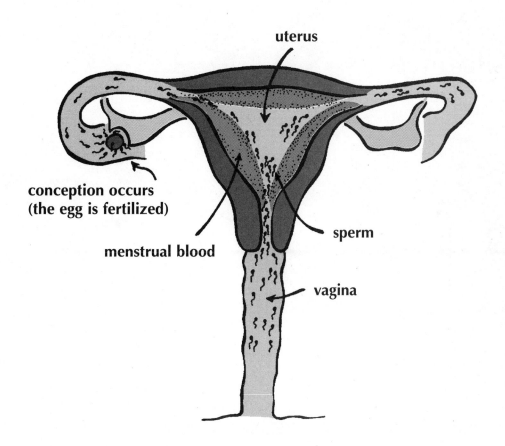

uterus

conception occurs
(the egg is fertilized)

menstrual blood

sperm

vagina

The fertilized egg travels through the Fallopian tube to the uterus. There it becomes implanted within the layers of blood that nourish it.

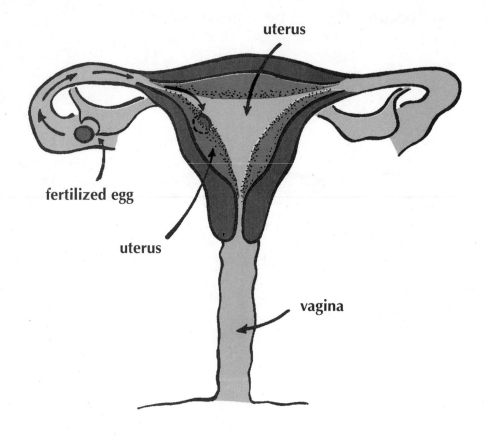

A baby begins to grow inside the woman's uterus. The layers of blood, instead of being lost, are used to nourish the growing embryo. (An unborn child is called an embryo for the first 2 months.) The woman misses her period and discovers she is **pregnant!**

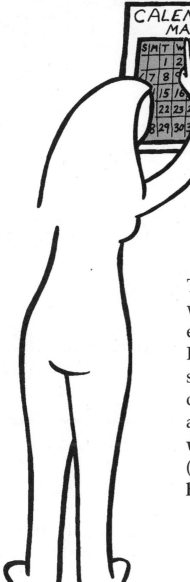

Timing Is Important

Timing is important because **conception** will only occur when a sperm meets an egg within about 24 hours after **ovulation**. However, sperm can remain active for several days inside the uterus waiting for ovulation to occur and an egg to become available for fertilization. This means **a woman can actually become pregnant** (if ovulation occurs) **up to four days after having sexual intercourse.**

HOW THE BABY GROWS

Drawings are actual size.

Pregnancy is usually *counted* from the first day of the last menstrual period. However, pregnancy *actually begins* with **conception,** which occurs within a day of **ovulation,** or about 14 days after the first day of the last period.

Therefore, at 4-1/2 weeks of pregnancy, the baby is usually only about 2 weeks along.

**4-1/2 weeks
(1 month)**

The heart starts beating. The embryo is now about 1/5-inch long. The woman has just missed her menstrual period for the first time. She thinks she might be pregnant.

**9 weeks
(2 months)**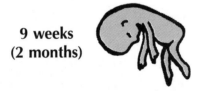

Now the baby is called a *fetus*, not an *embryo*. It is basically fully formed. All the parts of a full-term baby are present. The fetus is just over an inch long.

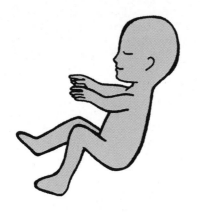

**13-1/2 weeks
(3 months)**

The fetus is about 2-1/2 to 3 inches long. Eyes are closed.

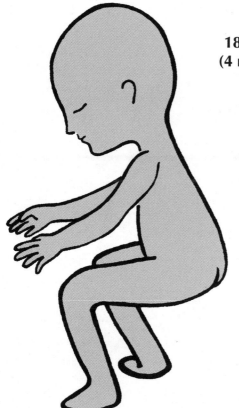

**18 weeks
(4 months)**

Arms and hands are fully formed, with fingernails. The fetus is about 6 inches long. It begins to drink several ounces of amniotic fluid every day.

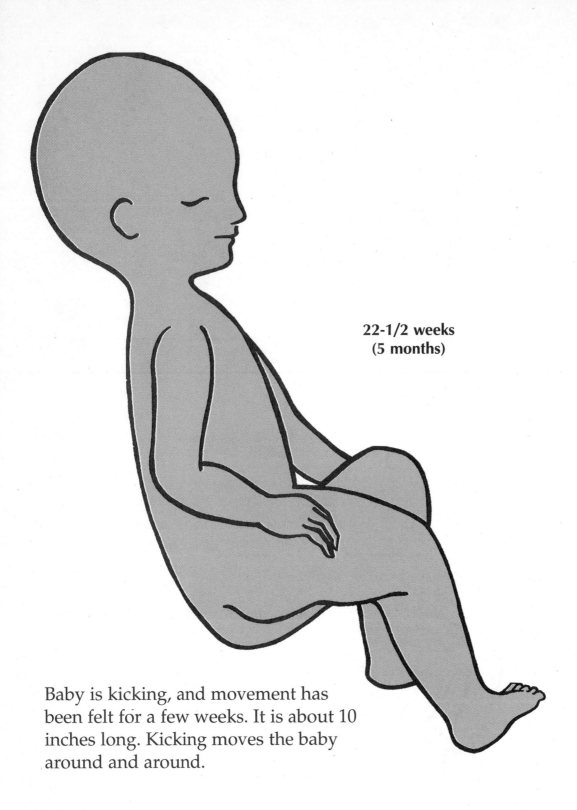

**22-1/2 weeks
(5 months)**

Baby is kicking, and movement has
been felt for a few weeks. It is about 10
inches long. Kicking moves the baby
around and around.

There is less space for the child. It is now over 12 inches long. The baby is very thin. It gains only 1/3 of its birth weight in the first 6 months of pregnancy. Now the baby probably weighs about 2-1/2 pounds.

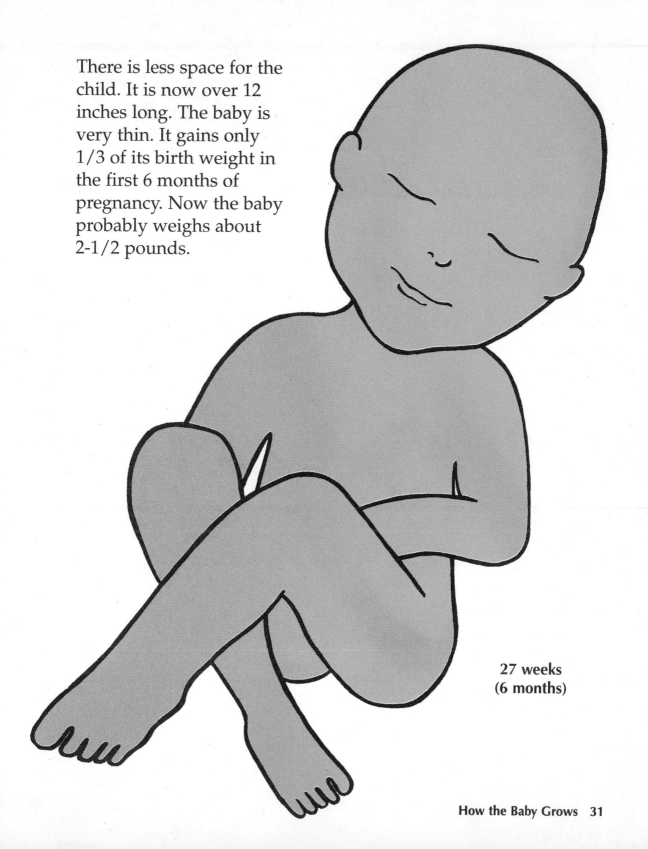

27 weeks
(6 months)

The fetus is usually over 13 inches long.

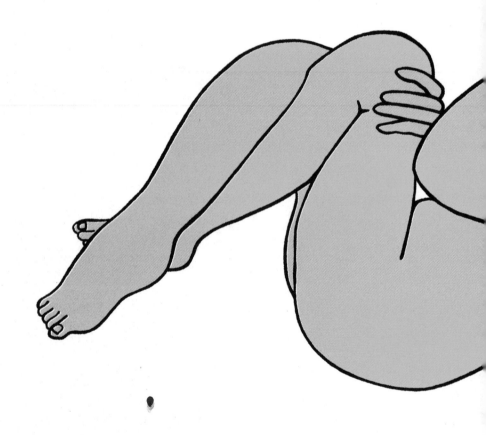

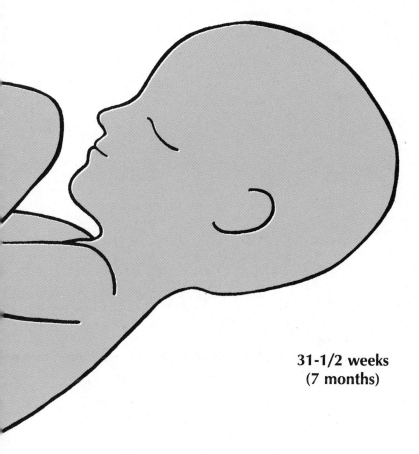

**31-1/2 weeks
(7 months)**

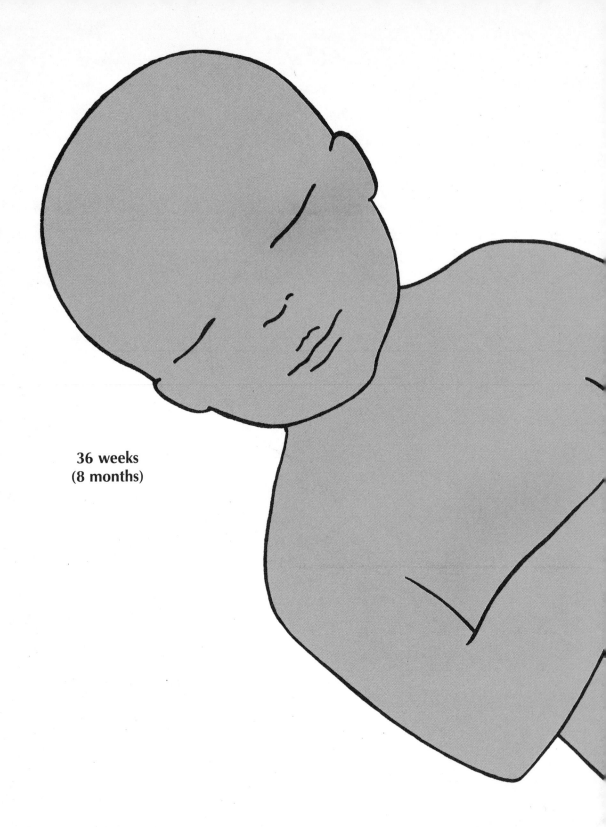

**36 weeks
(8 months)**

The fetus is usually between 15 and 17 inches long. During this month, brain cells form more rapidly than at any other time in a person's whole life. A good diet for the mother that includes enough protein is especially important.

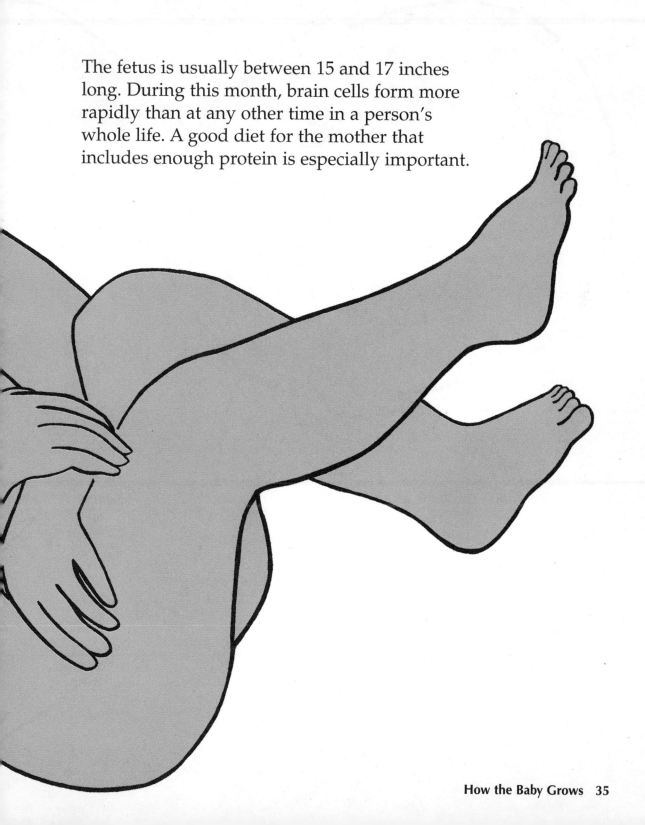

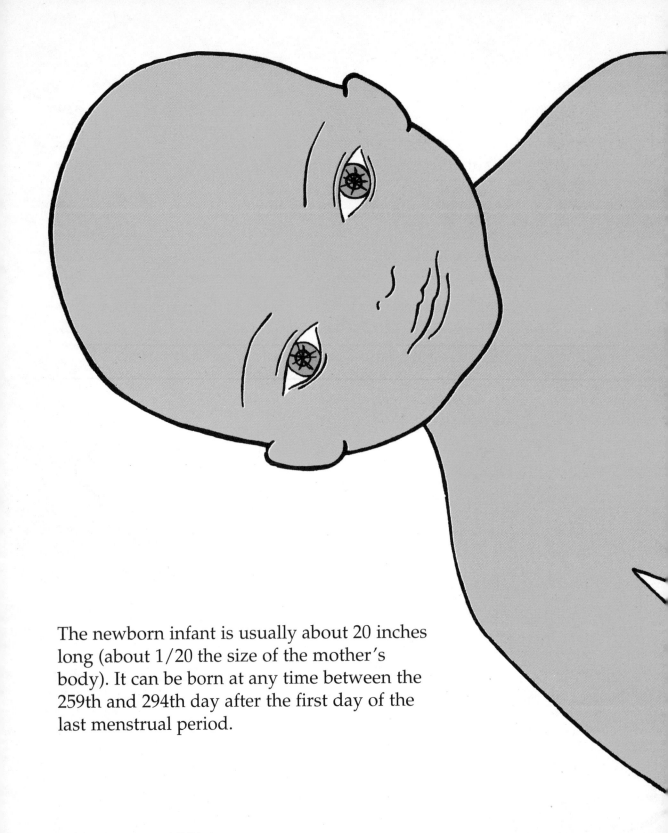

The newborn infant is usually about 20 inches long (about 1/20 the size of the mother's body). It can be born at any time between the 259th and 294th day after the first day of the last menstrual period.

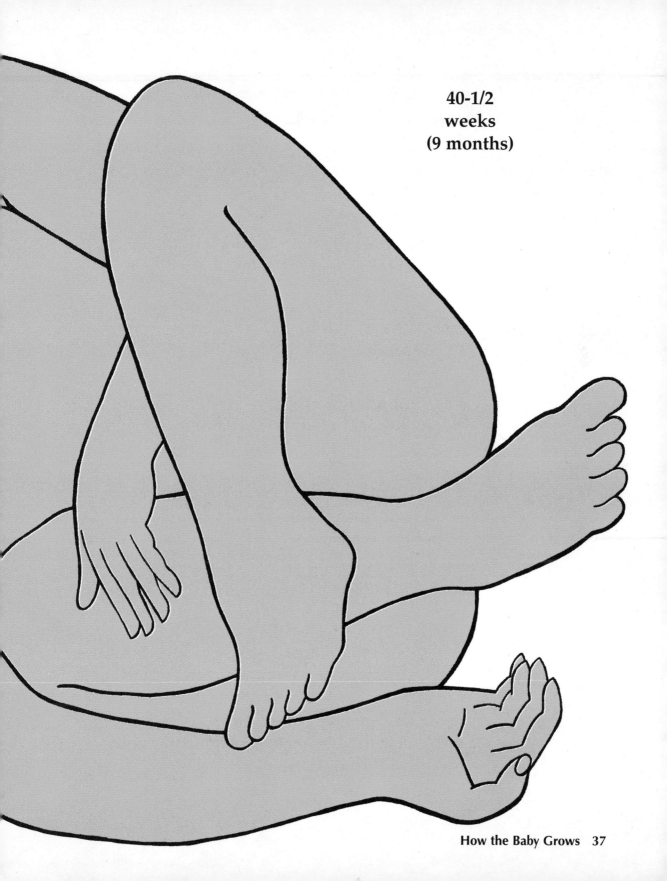

40-1/2
weeks
(9 months)

WHERE THE BABY GROWS

We have seen *how* the baby grows. In order to understand pregnancy, labor and birth, you must also understand *where* the baby is growing and *what parts* of the mother's body are affected.

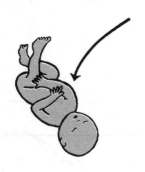

The **baby** can see, hear, and is recording memories even before it is born.

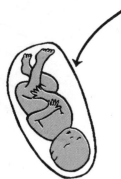

The **amnion** (water bag). The baby is inside a **bag of waters** called the **amnion**. It is thin and made of layers. It is filled with amniotic fluid and the baby.

A good diet helps keep the amnion strong and from breaking too soon.

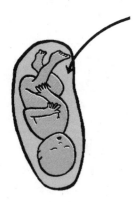

Amniotic fluid is often called the *waters*. This is the clear, salty fluid that surrounds the baby inside the amnion. From the fourth month on, the baby drinks several ounces of amniotic fluid every day. It is part of the baby's food before birth. This fluid helps to cushion and protect the baby during pregnancy.

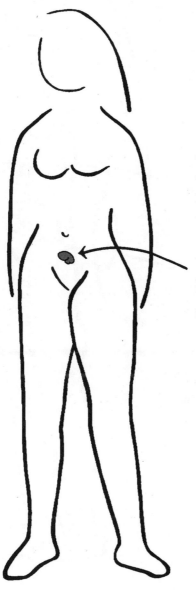

Another bag surrounds the amnion. It is a very powerful muscle-bag called the **uterus** or **womb.**

When a woman is not pregnant, the uterus is about the size of a small pear.

During pregnancy, the uterus grows to about 20 times its nonpregnant size and becomes very strong. This strong muscle is shaped like a bag and holds and protects the baby.

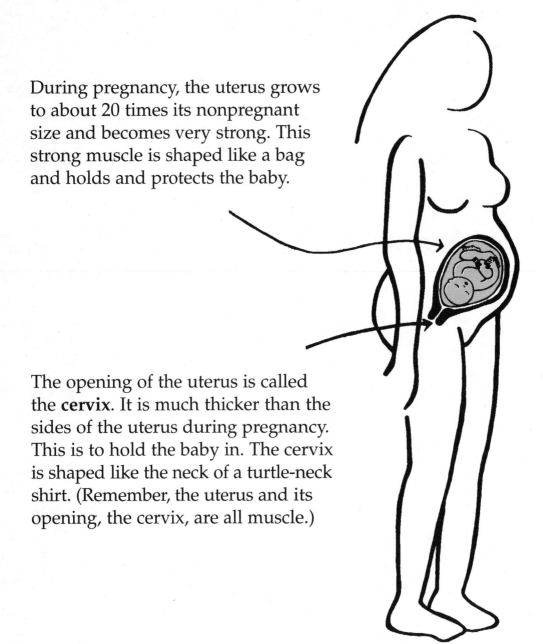

The opening of the uterus is called the **cervix**. It is much thicker than the sides of the uterus during pregnancy. This is to hold the baby in. The cervix is shaped like the neck of a turtle-neck shirt. (Remember, the uterus and its opening, the cervix, are all muscle.)

The amnion is connected to the inside of the uterus by the **placenta**. The word placenta comes from a Latin word meaning *flat cake*. The placenta is flat and round.

The placenta is the baby's life-support system. Through the placenta the baby receives food and oxygen from the mother's blood. Waste from the baby's body passes into the mother's blood through the placenta. The placenta can be compared to the filter on a fish tank.

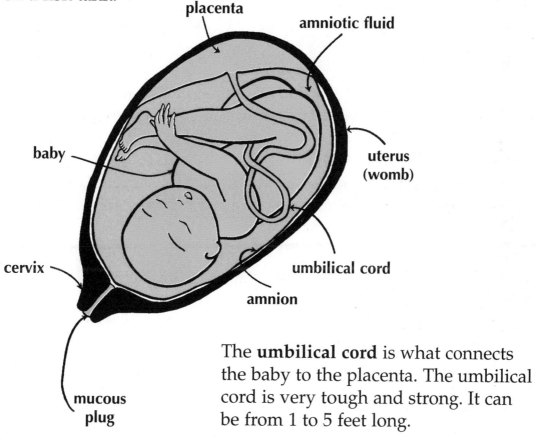

The **umbilical cord** is what connects the baby to the placenta. The umbilical cord is very tough and strong. It can be from 1 to 5 feet long.

The opening of the cervix is sealed with a thick **mucous plug** from the beginning of pregnancy. This protects the baby and prevents any contamination from getting in the uterus.

WHAT HAPPENS INSIDE THE WOMAN'S BODY AS THE BABY GROWS?

(1) The **abdomen** is the middle part of your body. The abdomen contains the stomach, intestines, liver and other organs.

(2) The **stomach** is a special muscular bag in the abdomen. The food you eat digests there so your body can use it.

(3) The **intestines** are the long, long tubes that carry food from the stomach through the body. Solid wastes (bowel movements) pass out of your body through your intestines.

(4) Above the stomach is the **liver**. The liver helps your body get good use from the food you eat. The liver also helps your body get rid of poisons, drugs or anything toxic in your food.

(5) Above the abdomen is the **diaphragm**. The diaphragm is a muscular wall that separates the abdomen from the chest area.

(6) The **heart** is in the chest. The heart is the muscle that pumps blood throughout your body.

(7) The **uterus** lies at the bottom part of the abdomen.

Before Pregnancy

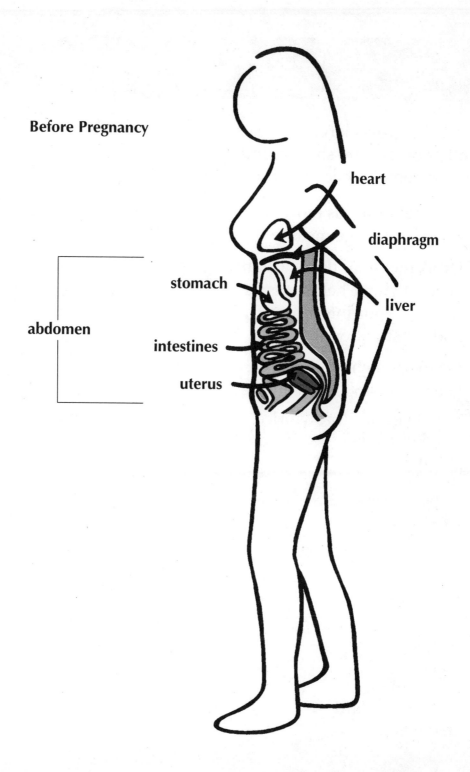

heart

diaphragm

stomach

liver

abdomen

intestines

uterus

Where Do the Stomach and Other Organs Go during Pregnancy?

As the baby grows larger and larger, the stomach, intestines, liver and other organs are shoved and squished *up* and *back.* They have much less room. It becomes especially important to:

- **Eat smaller meals more frequently.** There is just not enough room for a large meal to digest well.

- **Drink plenty of fluids.** (Eight large glasses of water each day is best.) Water helps keep the food you've eaten moving through your intestines. This helps to prevent indigestion and constipation.

- **Eat foods high in fiber.** These foods absorb water and help keep your stools soft and regular. Some high-fiber foods are:

  whole grains (brown rice, whole-grain cereals, pastas
      and breads)
  beans
  salads
  other vegetables
  raw fruits

- **Don't eat fatty foods.** They are hard to digest. These foods might give you indigestion during pregnancy. They take longer to digest than other foods. Some high-fat foods are:

  fatty, oily or fried foods
  pastries
  nuts
  nut butters
  butter and lard
  red meats

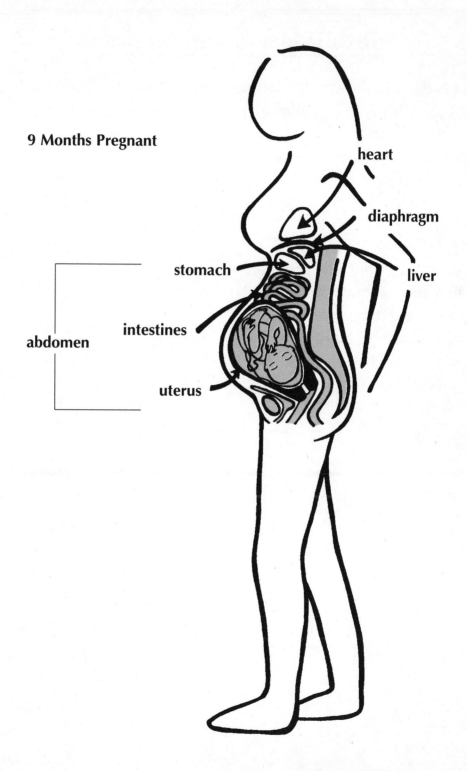

9 Months Pregnant

heart

diaphragm

stomach

liver

abdomen

intestines

uterus

The Bladder during Pregnancy

The **bladder** is the small triangle-shaped bag that holds urine. In a woman's body it lies above and behind the *pubic bone* and in front of the *uterus.*

As the baby grows in the *uterus,* the uterus and baby get heavier and heavier. The bladder gets more and more squashed against the pubic bone.

By the ninth month of pregnancy, the bladder is squashed completely flat against the pubic bone. The baby's head is usually on one side of the bladder. The pubic bone is on the other side.

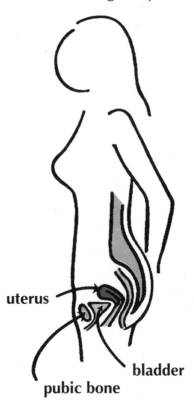

Before Pregnancy

uterus

bladder

pubic bone

This puts a lot of pressure *on* the bladder, which feels just like pressure *in* the bladder. In other words, the weight of the baby on the bladder makes a woman feel like she must urinate. But when she goes to the toilet, often only a few drops come out.

She feels the weight of the baby pressing the bladder against the pubic bone. This feels just like a full bladder.

And whenever she walks or runs, the baby bounces again and again against her bladder. This often makes her head for the toilet.

9 Months Pregnant

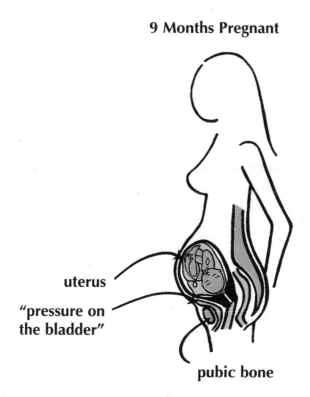

uterus

"pressure on
the bladder"

pubic bone

The Muscle of the Pelvic Floor
(The "P.C." Muscle)

The P.C. muscle goes from the pubic bone in front to the **tail bone** or **coccyx** in back. These two bones give the muscle its full name, the **pubococcygeus muscle,** or **P.C.** for short. It has also been called the **Kegel muscle,** after Dr. Arnold Kegel, who did a lot of research about it.

Bladder Control

The P.C. muscle is shaped like a hammock. It forms the floor of the pelvis. In women it supports the bladder, uterus, vagina and rectum. A strong P.C. muscle gives you good bladder and bowel control. If you pass urine when you cough, laugh, sneeze, hiccup or burp, you probably have a weak P.C. muscle.

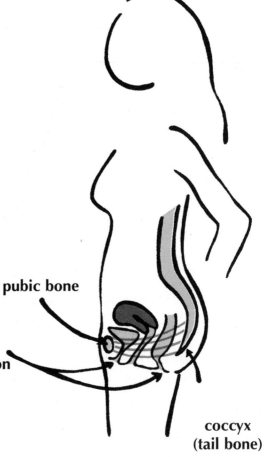

pubic bone

P.C. muscle
in good condition

The urethra, vagina
and rectum pass directly
through the P.C. muscle

coccyx
(tail bone)

A strong P.C. muscle keeps you from urinating or moving your bowels when you don't want to. A weak P.C. muscle leads to lack of bladder or bowel control (incontinence).

A weak muscle cannot support the organs of the pelvic area. The uterus can sag and the urethra and rectum lose support.

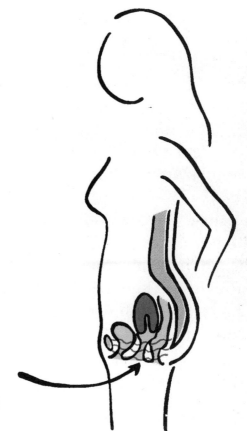

P.C. muscle in poor shape (Urine may leak from your bladder at times.)

The P.C. Muscle in Pregnancy

Pregnancy puts a lot of pressure on the P.C. muscle. The P.C. muscle helps to support the growing uterus and baby. It also controls the extra urine you have when you are pregnant.

The vagina goes right through the P.C. muscle. During the birth of a child, the P.C. muscle gets stretched a lot. Women with a strong P.C. muscle do not have problems following birth. A strong P.C. muscle quickly snaps back into shape. But women with a weak P.C. muscle may lose bladder control following birth.

Fortunately, you can exercise the P.C. muscle during pregnancy. This can help to make it strong. A strong P.C. muscle will give you good bladder control both during pregnancy and after giving birth.

P.C. muscle in good shape during pregnancy.

How to Exercise the P.C. Muscle

You can exercise the P.C. muscle by tightening up as if to hold your urine. Slowly count to five and then relax. You can practice while sitting on the toilet. Practice stopping and starting your flow of urine.

After getting used to the exercise, you can do it anywhere, anytime (while walking, driving, cooking, standing in lines and so forth). No one will know you are doing it!

Do the P.C. exercise in sets of five or 10 at a time throughout the day. During pregnancy do between 10 and 20 sets of these each day.

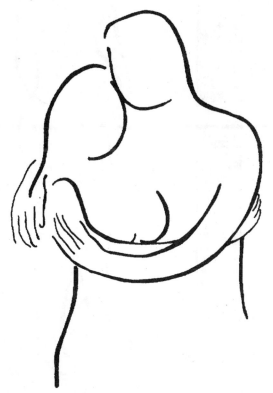

Men have P.C. muscles, too. A strong P.C. muscle can give *anyone* good bladder control, whether young or old.

Sexual Response

A woman who develops a strong P.C. muscle may find that sex gets better for herself and her partner. With a strong P.C. muscle your vagina is naturally tighter. A tight vagina gives you and your partner more stimulation during intercourse. This can bring you both a better sex life.

BLOOD VOLUME

The amount of blood in a woman's body increases during pregnancy as much as 40%. This is natural and normal. But what does it do to her body?

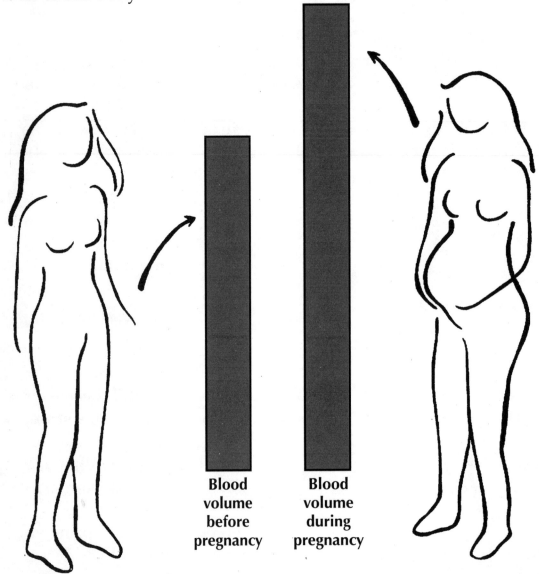

Blood volume before pregnancy

Blood volume during pregnancy

Varicose Veins, Hemorrhoids and Fatigue

The extra blood volume can cause your blood vessels to swell. Circulation (movement of the blood) can slow down. Varicose veins (swollen veins) may appear in your legs. You may get hemorrhoids (swollen veins in the rectum). And you may feel tired much of the time.

What can you do? Exercise!

Exercise at least 20 minutes every day when you are pregnant. Low-intensity aerobic exercise like walking is best. Regular exercise makes your body make **more channels through which the blood can flow**! This cuts down swelling in your veins. It improves circulation. And exercise can increase your energy level.

Aerobic exercises are those that are steady and nonstop. They make your heart beat faster. Good aerobic exercises during pregnancy include brisk walking, swimming and outdoor or stationary bicycling. Don't run or jog or do any exercise that bounces your body. Don't let yourself get too tired. It is also important to wear light clothing. Don't overheat your body when you exercise during pregnancy.

It is wise to check with your doctor before beginning any program of exercise while pregnant. Stop any exercise that causes vaginal bleeding, spotting or cramping. Report any such symptoms to your doctor right away.

Position for Sleeping

When a woman is pregnant and sleeps or lies flat on her back, the weight of the baby, and the uterus, and the waters puts pressure on a major body vein (vena cava). This slows down the flow of blood throughout the entire body. This can contribute to abnormal swelling of the legs (edema) and varicose veins. **Labor is slowed down in this position.**

A woman with a very large baby or twins can pass out (faint) if made to lie on her back. If the movement of blood throughout the body is slowed down, you will feel tired, even after sleeping.

Wrong Position

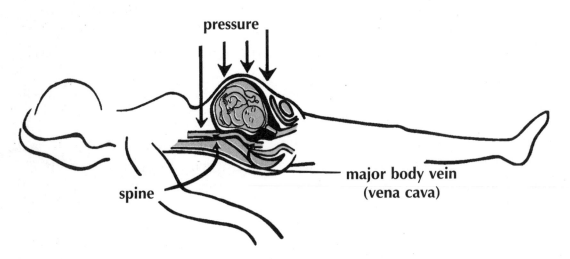

pressure

spine

major body vein
(vena cava)

Any side position is O.K. for sleeping or resting. Lying on your side helps your blood move well throughout your body. This helps you get a better rest.

Right Position

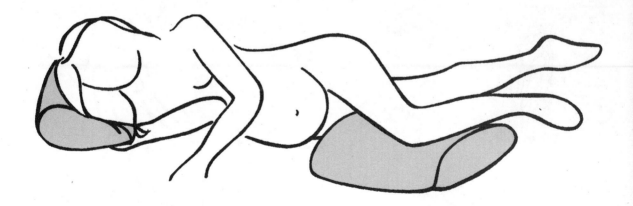

A Good Diet Is Important!

Some people believe that a baby will take whatever it needs from the mother's body. This is just not true! **The foods a pregnant woman eats every day are the foods that build the baby's body.**

The special needs of the growing baby make it important that the mother's diet be excellent. Through her diet and the care she takes, she gives the child the gift of a poorly or well-formed body.

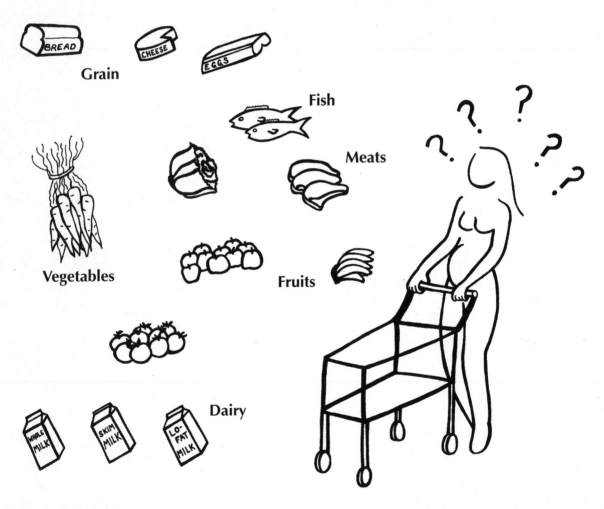

Grain

Fish

Meats

Vegetables

Fruits

Dairy

Junk Foods Cannot Build a Healthy Body for the Baby

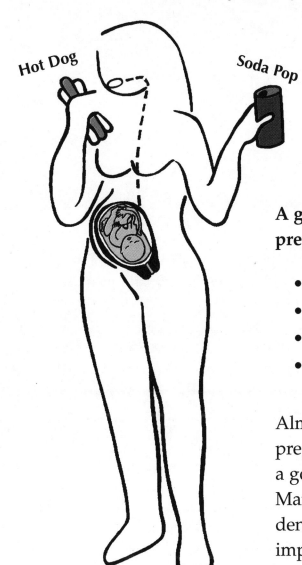

Hot Dog

Soda Pop

A poor diet during pregnancy can help cause <u>birth defects</u>.

A good diet during pregnancy can help ensure:

- A normal, healthy, strong baby
- An easy, comfortable pregnancy
- An easier labor and birth
- A healthy, happy mother

Almost every complaint of pregnancy can be resolved through a good diet and proper exercise. Many complaints disappear suddenly as soon as the diet is improved.

What to Eat

(See worksheet on page 119.)

A well-balanced diet means eating a good variety of foods:

- fruits
- vegetables
- grains
- dairy products (milk and cheeses)
- protein foods (meats, fish, eggs, nuts or beans)

It is important to eat foods from each of these groups every day. This helps you make sure that the baby gets all the nutrients it needs for a healthy, well-formed body.

Foods lose many important nutrients when they are processed. For instance, a potato contains more food value than potato chips. Brown rice contains more food value than white rice or puffed rice. Whole-wheat or corn flour and whole-wheat bread or corn tortillas contain more food value than white flour and white bread or white flour tortillas.

Make simple foods at home from fresh ingredients as often as you can. Such home-made meals probably cost less and are better for you than most frozen or canned foods or meals prepared in restaurants.

Sweets and Fats

Sweets make a pregnant woman feel full. But they do not provide much food value for the growing child (or for mom, either). Eat less of these foods during pregnancy, or none at all!

- candies
- cookies
- cakes
- pastries

- butter
- lard
- cream
- cooking oils

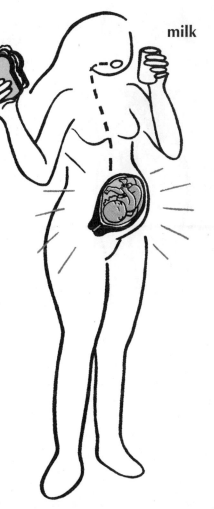

milk

healthy sandwich on
whole-wheat bread

Weight Gain

A healthy woman on a good diet gains about 25 to 35 pounds during pregnancy. However, if a pregnant woman gains the same amount of weight on *junk* foods, she can really be in trouble. The important thing is not how much weight is gained, but what *kinds* of food she is eating to gain it.

The Liver during Pregnancy

Red blood cells are always being made within your body. They live for about 120 days, and then they die. New red blood cells are always being made to take their place.

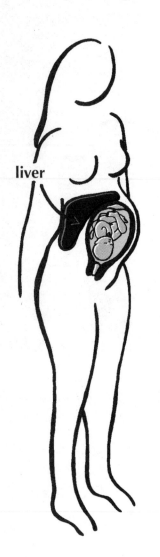

liver

Your liver collects all the dead red blood cells. It also collects any bits of strange chemicals or poisons you may have eaten, such as the chemical preservatives in some foods. Your liver gets rid of these things so your blood can stay clean and healthy. Your liver is working all the time to keep your blood clean.

During pregnancy, the baby's liver is still developing. It does not yet work very well. **Think of the number of times you have to change a baby's diaper after it is born! During pregnancy, all the baby's wastes get dumped into the mother's bloodstream every day, instead.** A pregnant woman's liver must work super-hard to help keep her blood clean.

DRUGS, ALCOHOL AND THE BABY

Drugs and alcohol are substances your liver works hard to clean out of your body. A pregnant woman's liver is *already* working very hard because of the pregnancy. Drugs or alcohol can just be too much. Her overworked liver may not be able to clean the drugs or alcohol out of her blood as fast or as well as it could before pregnancy. Because of this, drugs and alcohol may have a greater effect on a woman during pregnancy. The effect on each woman is different.

When you take drugs or alcohol during pregnancy they go straight to the baby. **The baby's developing liver cannot easily get these substances out of the baby's body. They tend to collect in the baby's body in *greater concentrations* than in the mother's body.**

> **Drugs and alcohol can damage the development of the baby's body during pregnancy.**

Drugs and alcohol during pregnancy can cause or contribute to a wide variety of birth defects in the child. **Don't use drugs or alcohol during pregnancy!**

Sometimes medications are necessary during pregnancy. But their benefits should be carefully weighed against the possible effect they could have on the unborn child.

Prevent Birth Defects

In 1988, one out of every 14 babies born in the United States was born with a birth defect (March of Dimes report).

You can reduce risks for your child.
During pregnancy, stay away from:

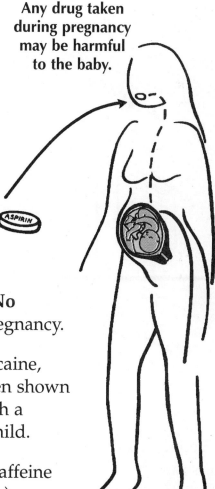

Any drug taken during pregnancy may be harmful to the baby.

(1) Drugs. These include nonprescription, over-the-counter medicines or home remedies, such as baking soda in water. Many prescription drugs, including sedatives and tranquilizers, are not safe during pregnancy.

(2) Smoking cigarettes, or anything at all. Tobacco in all forms.

(3) Alcohol, including beer and wine. **No** amount of alcohol is safe during pregnancy.

(4) Illegal drugs, such as marijuana, cocaine, crack, heroin and PCP. Each has been shown to create serious health risks for both a pregnant woman and her unborn child.

(5) Coffee, tea or anything containing caffeine (including cola drinks and chocolate).

(6) Bad eating habits.

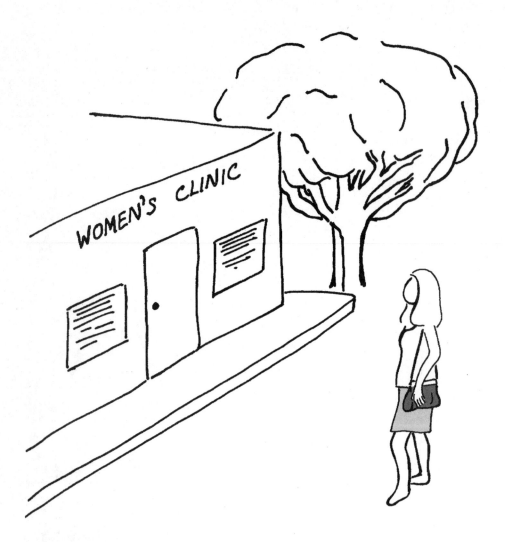

Prenatal care means regular visits to a doctor, midwife or clinic throughout pregnancy. The schedule of your visits will vary, but usually include:

—an overall physical exam;

This exam should be done early in pregnancy, usually within a week or two of learning you're pregnant. Your healthcare provider will:

- confirm your pregnancy
- check the state of your health
- discover any possible problems that need correction —or watching.

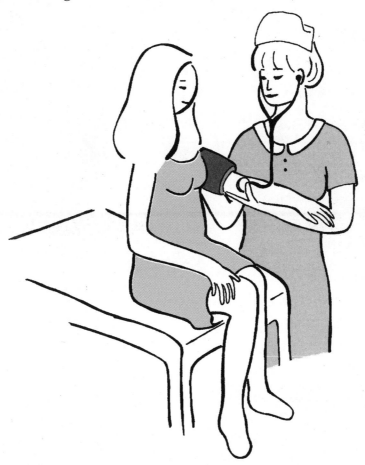

—regular monthly check-ups, up to the seventh month;

Your healthcare provider will:

- listen to the baby's heartbeat

- measure your uterus (from the outside) to check that your baby is growing normally

- check that you are gaining enough weight

- check your blood pressure and check samples of your blood (for anemia or infection)

- check your urine (for sugar, protein or infection)

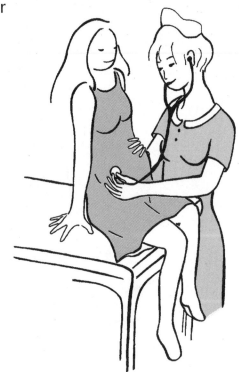

- examine your hands and feet for signs of abnormal swelling (edema)

- discuss any physical problems you may have been having

- try to answer your questions. (Be sure to write down any questions you may have before your check-up.)

—regular check-ups every 2 weeks in the eighth month, and once a week in the ninth month, until the baby is born.

Check-ups will be the same. But now your provider will check:

- the size and position of the baby
- your cervix (see page 40) to see if it is softening or thinning out.

Your cervix is hard and firm during pregnancy, but softens just before the baby is ready to be born. Some providers speak of the cervix as **green** when it is firm and **ripe** when it is soft. A soft, "ripe" cervix means the baby will soon be born!

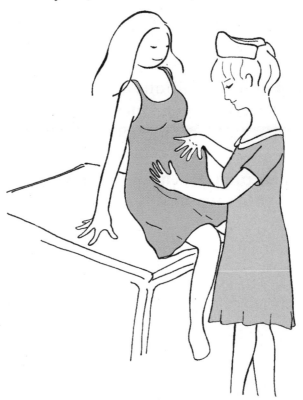

Prenatal Care Is Important

Regular prenatal check-ups can help your doctor or midwife discover and correct or prevent many problems such as:

- **anemia** (low levels of iron and oxygen in your blood)

- **gestational diabetes** (diabetes that only occurs during pregnancy)

- **pre-eclampsia** (a potentially dangerous condition signaled by high blood pressure, abnormal swelling and protein in the urine).

- **infections** (which can help make a baby come *too soon* or be *too small*).

These and other conditions are often easily corrected when discovered early in pregnancy. But, if left untreated, they can cause serious problems for you and your baby.

Start regular prenatal check-ups early in pregnancy. They help safeguard your own health and the health and well-being of your baby.

Labor—What Is It?

The uterus, the large muscle-bag that holds the baby, is thickest at the cervix (opening of the uterus) during pregnancy. The thick cervix helps hold the baby inside.

In order for the baby to come out, the thick cervix becomes thin and then opens wide enough for the baby to pass through.

This thinning (also called **effacing**) and opening of the cervix (**dilation**) occurs very gradually, little by little over a number of hours. The uterus tightens, pulling the cervix back just a little. Then it relaxes. The tightenings and relaxings of the uterus are **contractions of labor**. First the **contractions** make the cervix thin. Then they pull the cervix open so the baby can pass through.

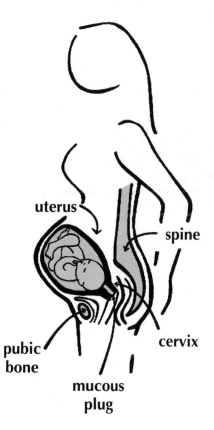

Before labor begins, cervix is thick.

uterus

spine

pubic bone

cervix

mucous plug

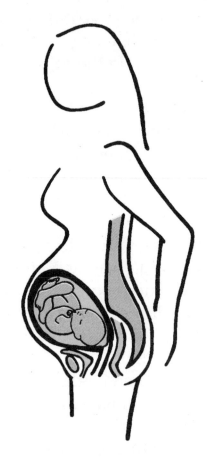

The whole **uterus** is a muscle. It simply rearranges itself during labor. It becomes thin and wide-open at the **cervix,** and thick at the other end. This is all there is to 90% of **labor.** This is the long **first stage of labor**, the rearranging of the **uterus** as it pulls the **cervix** open.

Cervix thinning but not open very much. Mucous plug is gone.

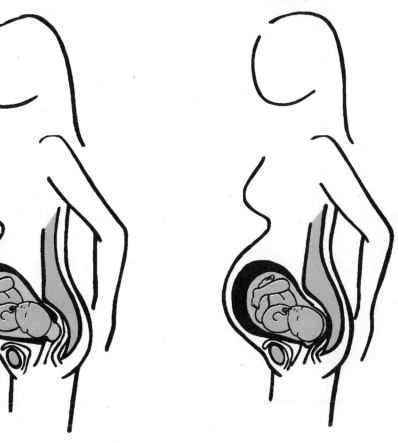

**First stage of labor
is complete.**

Cervix half-way open.

**Cervix fully open.
"Ready to push the baby out."**

All that's left is for **pushing contractions** to begin. Then the thick bottom end of the **uterus** begins pushing out the baby. (The short **second stage of labor.**)

Three Signs of Labor

1 **Loss of the mucous plug.** Also called the *bloody show*.

As the cervix begins to thin out and open up, the mucous plug falls away. It passes through the vagina and out of the body. Sometimes small bits of the inside of the cervix are pulled away with it. There may be blood with the mucous plug, from the inside edges of the cervix, where it was attached. When this happens, the loss of the mucous plug is called the *bloody show*. (It doesn't hurt when you lose the mucous plug.)

The loss of the mucous plug or bloody show is a sign that the cervix has begun to thin out and open up. So, it is a sign that *labor* has begun.

False Labor

Many women have "false labor" or many little practice contractions during the last month or two of pregnancy.

These small "practice" contractions are not real labor because the baby is not yet ready to be born. But, they can cause the cervix to thin out and even open up a little, as much as a month or more before real labor begins.

And so sometimes the mucous plug is lost (the bloody show is seen) weeks before real labor begins. If this happens, it can mean that real labor may be a little shorter. It is nothing to worry about. Tell your doctor or midwife, however, any time this sign of labor is seen.

You can also lose the mucous plug without noticing it, during one of your frequent trips to the toilet.

WARNING: If your pregnancy is less than 37 weeks along when you lose your mucous plug, **do not make love.** Sexual activity might make the baby come too soon. Wait until you get to 37 weeks, at least. Then it should be safe to make love all you want.

2 Contractions. (The uterus gets tight and relaxes again as it works to open up the cervix.)

The surest sign that labor has begun are regular contractions that do not go away, no matter what a woman is doing and no matter what position she is in.

Because "practice" contractions (false labor) are common, the best way to tell if these contractions are really labor is to walk around, take a warm shower, or otherwise change your position and activity. If the contractions turn off, it was probably "false labor."

But, if the contractions get stronger and closer together after changing your activity and position a few times, then you are probably in labor!

If you also pass blood or mucous from the vagina at this time, you can be sure you are in real labor.

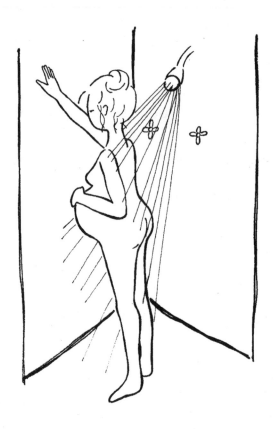

3 **Amnion (Bag of Waters) Breaks.** If the amnion (bag of waters) breaks at any time during pregnancy, call your healthcare provider to let him or her know. Contractions should begin within 12 to 24 hours from the time the amnion (bag of waters) breaks. Contractions may also begin right away.

It is wise to put a rubber sheet over your mattress, under your regular sheet, to protect the mattress in case the amnion (bag of waters) breaks while you're in bed.

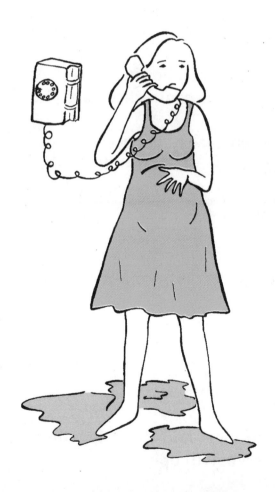

The Purpose of Contractions

First-Stage Labor

The whole purpose of contractions is to **dilate the cervix, to pull it open** so that the baby can come out. Every time you have a contraction, **relax** your vaginal area and the rest of your body. This can help the cervix to open as wide as it can.

Rest Periods

Remember, contractions of labor turn on and **off.** They allow a woman to **rest** between them. Contractions every 4 minutes mean only 15 contractions in an hour. And the closer together (and stronger!) the contractions are, the sooner the baby will be born!

Contractions of labor accelerate or speed up, much as a car gathers speed as you shift into higher gears. When contractions begin, they usually only last 30 seconds, and may be 20 minutes or more apart.

Gradually, the contractions get closer together—15 minutes apart, 10 minutes apart, 5 minutes apart—3 minutes apart.

Little by little, the contractions get longer—30 seconds long, 45 seconds long, 1 minute long, 1-1/2 minutes long. Sometimes, just before it's time to push out the baby, contractions may even be lasting 2 minutes!

The stronger and closer together the contractions get, the faster the cervix will open.

Dilation (Opening) of the Cervix

Drawings are actual size.

Your **work** is to **relax the rest of your body completely** while the uterus is working harder and faster to open the cervix. And it is **work.** It can take anywhere from 2 to 24 hours, or more, for the cervix of a normal healthy woman to open fully so that she is ready to push out the baby.

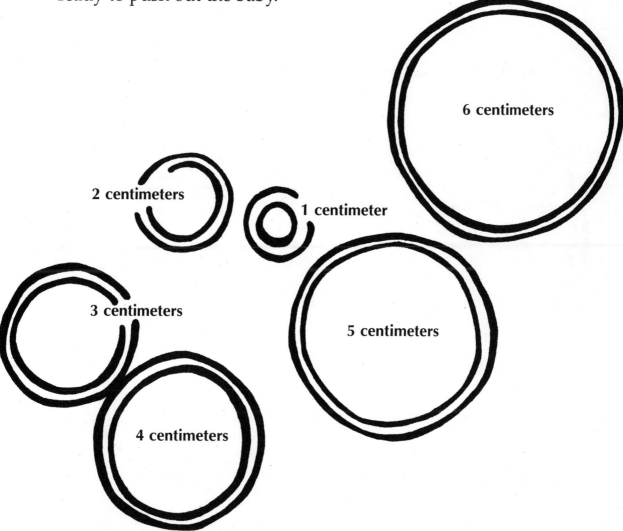

6 centimeters

2 centimeters

1 centimeter

3 centimeters

5 centimeters

4 centimeters

As soon as the cervix is open fully (to 10 centimeters) **the contractions ease up. They get shorter, further apart and less strong.** This is always a very welcome break. Just before full dilation, the contractions are very strong, very long and close together.

As soon as your cervix is open fully, you get to push out the baby. This is usually the most fun and exciting part for everyone!

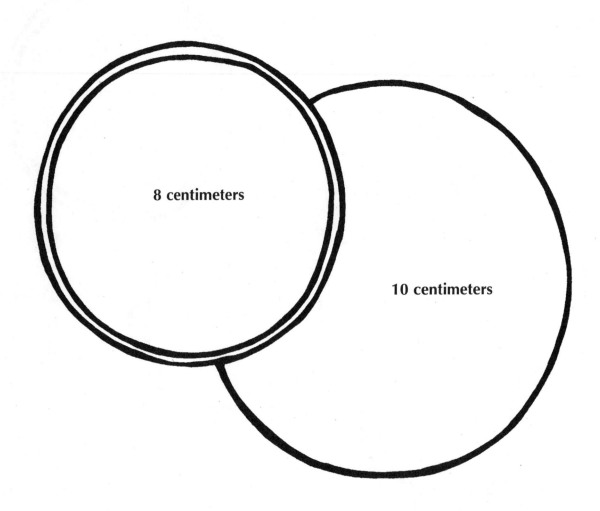

8 centimeters

10 centimeters

Vaginal Exams during First-Stage Labor

Doctor, nurse, or midwife's hand is shown checking how far the cervix has opened. The woman in labor is on her back—just for the vaginal exam.

The cervix has opened to about 3 centimeters. The amnion (bag of waters) has not yet broken.

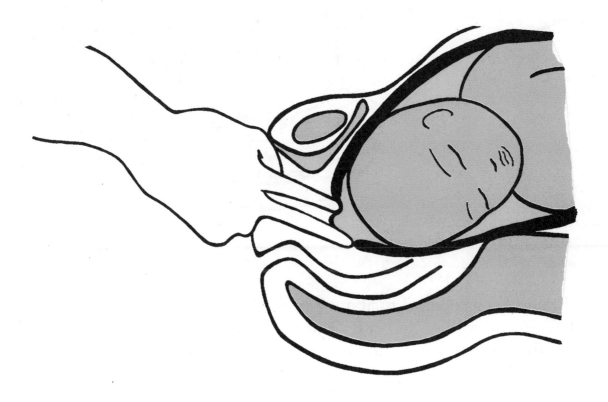

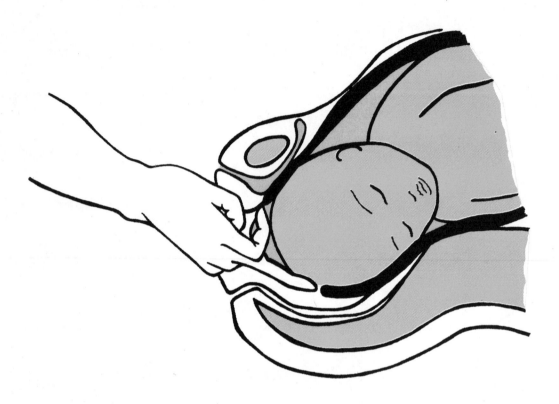

The cervix has opened to about 7 or 8 centimeters. The amnion (bag of waters) has not yet broken. The baby has moved down and the bladder and rectum are under a lot of pressure.

The cervix is fully open (dilated to 10 centimeters.) The baby's head has come *through* the cervix.

The amnion (bag of waters) has not yet broken. The rectum is squeezed flat against the bottom of the spine. The bladder is under a lot more pressure, too.

Now she's ready to **push out the baby!**

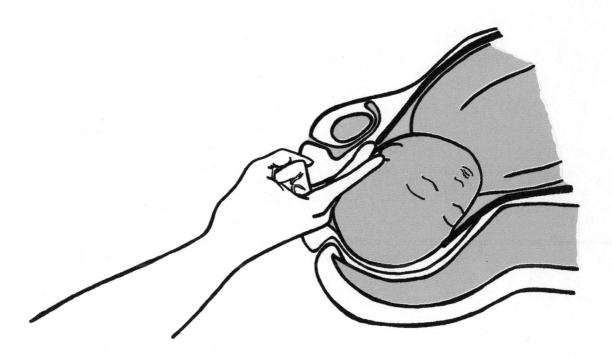

Transition

The word **transition** means **a period of change**. Transition in labor means the change in the action of the uterus, from **opening up the cervix** to **pushing out the baby**.

This is a major change for your body. Your blood circulation undergoes a major change. The blood concentrates in the area of the uterus.

Transition can be called the last 2 or 3 centimeters of dilation, when the cervix goes from 7 to 10 centimeters. Transition includes the whole time it takes for the contractions to change from *opening contractions* to *pushing contractions.*

Transition contractions are often very intense. They can be quite painful. It is good that transition is the shortest part of labor. Most of the time it lasts between 10 minutes and an hour. One half hour is about the average length of transition.

Transition is the change from . . .

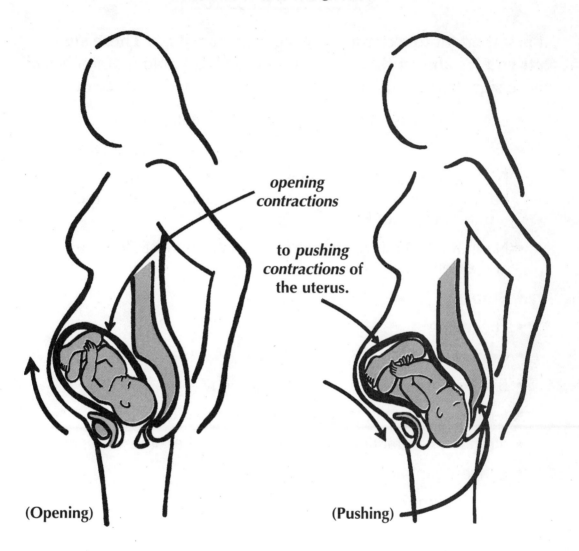

opening
contractions

to *pushing*
contractions of
the uterus.

(Opening)

(Pushing)

The lower part of the spine (tail bone or coccyx) becomes flexible.
It can straighten out to make more room for the baby as it passes
through the birth canal.

Signs of Transition

It is important to recognize the signs of transition. **These signs tell you it's almost time to push out the baby!** No woman has *all* these signs of transition. Most women have two or three of them.

- Legs or body trembling (caused by circulation changes)
- Hot or cold flashes (also caused by circulation changes)
- Feeling like having to have a bowel movement (pressure of the baby as it moves down, pressing the rectum against the bottom of the spine)
- Nausea or vomiting (depends on what you last ate, and when it was)
- Burping
- Hiccuping
- Confusion
- Bad disposition—you may feel grouchy
- Feeling of wanting to leave (wherever you are)
- Strongest contractions (contractions may become very painful)
- Longest contractions
- Contractions closest together (may be as close as 20 seconds apart)

An understanding **coach** is the *most* help during transition. Back rubs or pressure may feel good.

Remember, transition is a *very short* period. As soon as second-stage labor begins and you start to push out the baby, **the signs of transition disappear.** The excitement and work of pushing out the baby take over.

BIRTH: SECOND-STAGE LABOR

The **birth** of the baby—**pushing out the baby**—is called **second-stage labor**. It is much shorter than first-stage labor (dilation). Second-stage labor can take 20 minutes or less, or an hour or more. But it rarely takes longer than 2 hours.

Pushing can be hard work. But pushing in second-stage labor is a different kind of work from the work of relaxing through contractions in first-stage labor.

Pushing out a baby is not painful at all to most women. But there is a *lot of pressure* as the baby moves down and out. Some women are surprised to discover pleasant sensations in second-stage labor.

And pushing out a baby is always exciting and a big emotional thrill.

Two groups of muscles work to push out a baby. The uterus works by itself. It pushes every time it contracts. But you push with your abdominal (stomach) muscles to help the uterus.

Second-Stage Labor

Pushing Out the Baby

Mother is supported by her coach, or many pillows, while pushing. Special beds or delivery tables can help you find a good position for pushing.

Here is one good position for pushing, *a modified squatting position.*

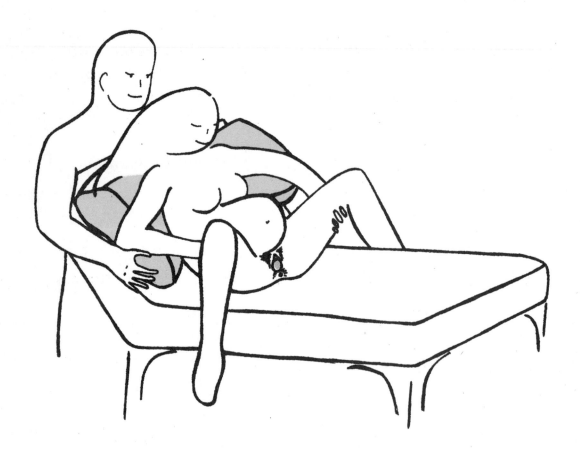

You help the uterus by pushing with your abdominal (stomach) muscles.

The uterus pushes all by itself.

It can take both the uterus and the woman pushing with her abdominal muscles, to push out a baby.

While both the uterus and the abdominal muscles are pushing, the baby moves down a little. Between contractions, when both muscles relax, the baby slips back a bit. Pushing is a "2 down, 1 back, 2 down, 1 back" kind of thing. After a while the baby's head will start to crown. This means you can see the baby's head in the vaginal opening. The vaginal opening forms a "crown" around the baby's head. Crowning is when the baby stays right there and doesn't slip back anymore.

Next—the baby is *out!*

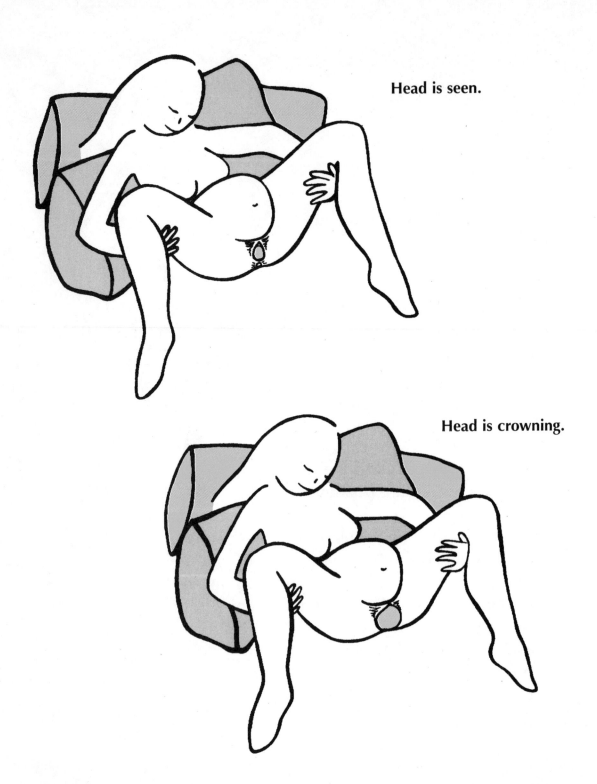

Head is seen.

Head is crowning.

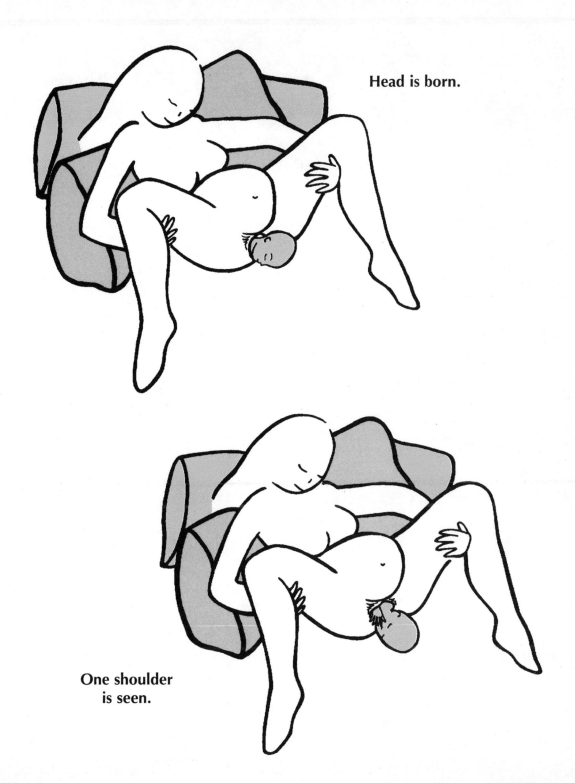

Head is born.

**One shoulder
is seen.**

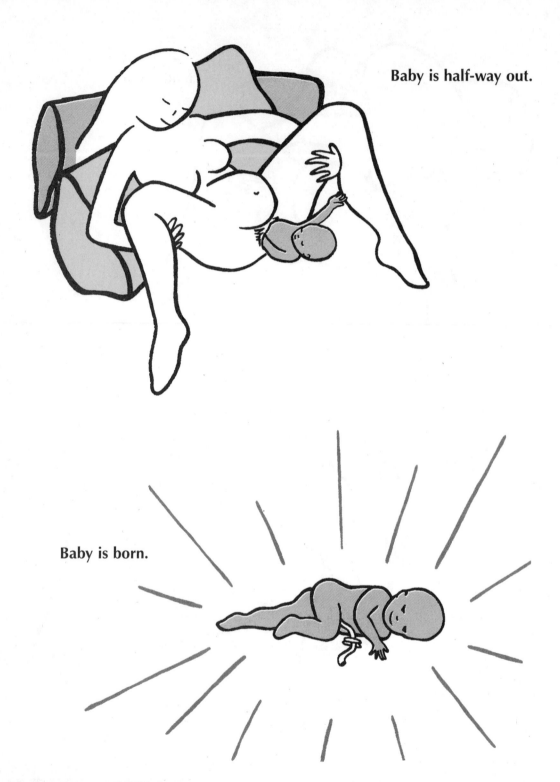

Baby is half-way out.

Baby is born.

Pushing Out the "Afterbirth"

Third stage is the last stage of labor. It is the shortest stage of labor. Third stage can take less than 15 minutes. But sometimes it takes longer for the placenta to separate from the inside of the uterus.

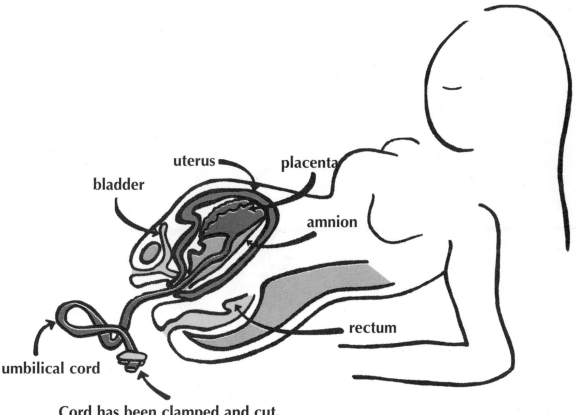

uterus

placenta

bladder

amnion

rectum

umbilical cord

Cord has been clamped and cut.

The placenta separates from the inside of the uterus.

In **third-stage labor** you push out the **afterbirth** (placenta, umbilical cord and amnion). You will feel the uterus contract a few more times. Push with the uterus, using your abdominal muscles, just as you did in second-stage labor when you pushed out the *baby*. (But it's much easier to push out the afterbirth.)

The "Afterbirth"

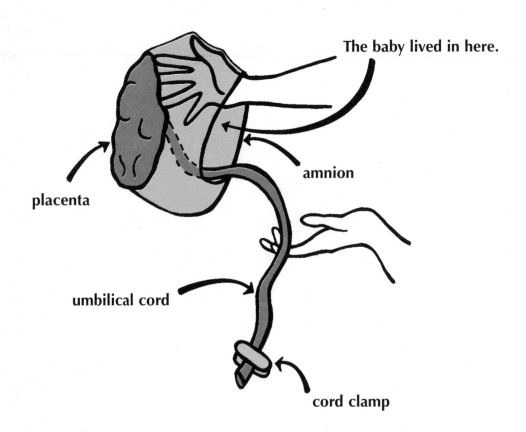

The baby lived in here.

amnion

placenta

umbilical cord

cord clamp

The bladder and rectum have been stretched out of shape by the birth of the child.

The large uterus sags. It is empty now that you have pushed out the afterbirth.

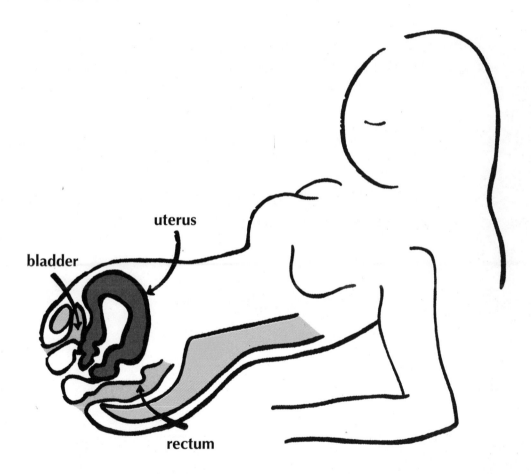

uterus

bladder

rectum

Massage the Uterus

The part of the uterus where the placenta was attached is full of open blood vessels. You will bleed freely after the placenta separates from the uterus.

How can you keep from bleeding too much? Gently rub or massage the uterus after the placenta comes out. This makes the uterus *contract* and cuts down the bleeding as the uterus tightens up.

How to Massage the Uterus

Gently rub the whole lower abdomen, below the navel. When something gets hard, keep rubbing that. It's the *uterus.*
Keep it "hard as a billiard ball and below the navel" for the first day after the baby is born. Rub the uterus every 15 minutes or so.

Between massages the uterus will relax. Try to keep it contracted into a hard ball, and *below the navel.* This helps to keep you from bleeding too much after the baby is born.

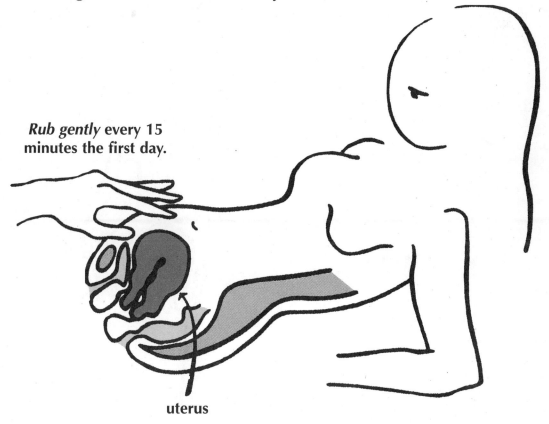

Rub gently every 15 minutes the first day.

uterus

Keep it "hard as a billiard ball and below the navel."

Getting Back to Normal

It takes about 6 weeks for the uterus, bladder and rectum of most women to return to their normal shapes after childbirth. The inside of the uterus, where the placenta was attached, will be healing. Nothing should enter the vagina until this healing is complete. Don't have sexual intercourse or use tampons until your after-birth bleeding has stopped. This can take from 2 to 6 weeks.

5 days after the birth

uterus

bladder

rectum

Breastfeeding

If you **breastfeed** the baby soon after it is born, and often in the first few days, a hormone will be released in your body. This hormone helps keep the uterus contracted and protects you from too much bleeding after the birth.

Breastfeeding also helps you get your figure back after childbirth. But don't try to diet. While you breastfeed, keep eating an excellent, well-balanced diet. This helps you make good-quality milk. (See worksheet on page 119.)

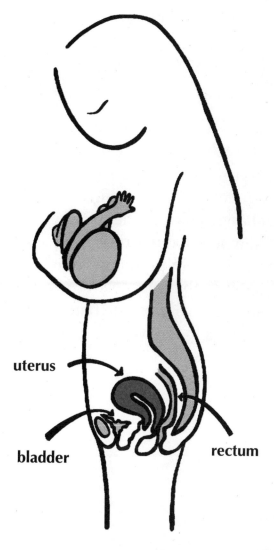

2 weeks after the birth

uterus

bladder

rectum

A new baby needs to be kept warm, to eat and to sleep. The baby will spend most of the first week sleeping. Most babies will wake to nurse every 2 or 3 hours, nurse for about 30 minutes or so, and then go back to sleep. Very sleepy babies can be gently awakened and encouraged to nurse (in the daytime) if they have slept at least 3 hours. This can help the baby sleep for longer periods of time at night.

Appearance

Normal newborns may look a bit wrinkled and puffy after all the squeezing and pushing of labor and birth. Eyes are blue-gray but change color in the coming months. So will the baby's skin. All newborns, regardless of race, appear pink-skinned at birth. Darker skin pigments take hours or days to develop. The skin of a new baby may seem to be peeling off within the first week or so, especially on the hands and feet. This is just a protective coating that covers the baby's skin before birth. It becomes dry and rubs off.

Rooming-In

After giving birth in a hospital or birth center, it is best if you and the baby can stay together at all times. This is called *rooming-in*. Rooming-in permits you to breastfeed and to respond directly to your baby's needs. While you get to know your baby, your baby learns to nurse, to feel secure and to trust you. A newborn can see, hear, smell, taste and is especially sensitive to touch.

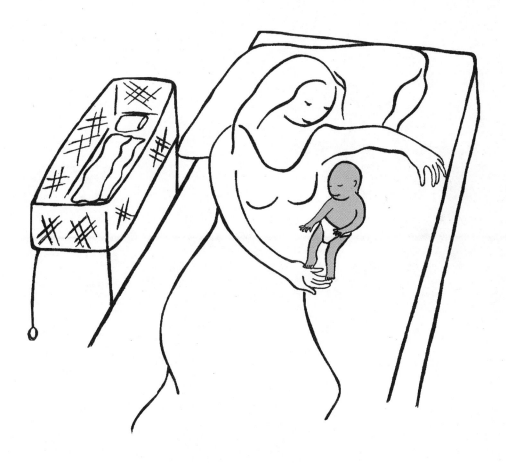

The Cord

The cord, which has been clamped and cut, should be kept clean and dry. The place where baby and cord meet should be swabbed with alcohol twice a day until the cord becomes completely dry. No oils should be used in this area. And no baths should be given until the cord falls off. (The baby can be wiped clean with a damp cloth until then.) The cord will fall off in 7 to 10 days or so. What's left is the navel (belly button).

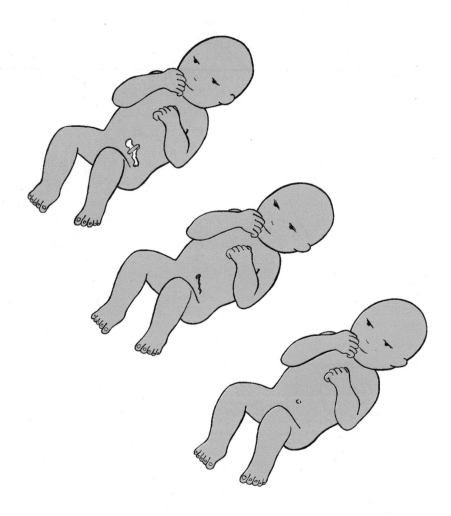

Bowel Movements

The baby's first bowel movements are black and sticky, like thick tar. They stain cloth diapers, no matter how many times you wash or bleach them. The loose, shapeless stools of a breastfed newborn usually appear by the end of the first week.

Weight Loss

Most babies lose a few ounces the first week. They are usually gaining weight again within 7 to 9 days. Babies whose mothers received drugs during labor and birth may suck less well and less often. They may lose more weight than babies whose mothers received no drugs. Frequent breastfeeding from the hour (or day) of birth cuts down on newborn weight loss. It also helps a new mother's breastmilk "come in."

Breastfeeding

True breastmilk doesn't appear within a new mother's breasts for 3 or 4 days. Before that time her breasts contain **colostrum.** Colostrum is much higher in protein than breastmilk. It is designed to protect the tiny newborn from disease. Colostrum has been called **"nature's vaccine"** because it begins to protect the baby with the first feeding.

There is nothing a new baby can be fed that is more important to its health and well-being than colostrum. If you give the baby a bottle (of *anything*) within the first few weeks you may confuse the baby and create problems with breastfeeding. Nursing at a breast is more work than sucking from a bottle. When babies learn the easier task of sucking from a bottle, they sometimes reject the breast.

Jaundice

A new baby's liver is young. It is hard for it to clean all the wastes from its blood. (During pregnancy, the placenta and the mother's liver kept the baby's blood clean.) When a newborn's liver cannot keep the bloodstream clean, the baby's skin may get a bit yellow. This is called *jaundice*.

Almost half of all normal newborns show some signs of jaundice. It can start from the second to the fourth day of life. Most of the time the jaundice is gone by the end of the first week and causes no problem. But, **jaundice that appears within the first 24 hours or after the first week could be harmful to the baby. If your baby looks yellow on these days, call your doctor right away.** And, if your baby ever looks very yellow or if the white part of her eyes becomes yellow, she should be checked by a doctor, just to be safe.

The Baby's Bed

New babies seem to sleep well on a smooth, firm surface. Raise the level of the baby's mattress 2 inches higher at the head than at the foot. This may protect the baby from harmful breathing problems. And put your baby to sleep on her back, not on her belly. This also helps her to breathe well and can prevent some cases of SIDS (sudden infant death syndrome).

Emotional Let-Down (Blues)

After all the months of waiting and getting ready, the baby has come. Many mothers are thrilled. But many new mothers can feel just the opposite—empty, numb, sad or a bit "lost." You can feel this sort of let-down after other major life events for which you have planned and prepared. The big day comes, and then it's over. The excitement and waiting that had filled your days are gone. It is common (and natural) to feel "let down" or "blue."

Your body needs time to get over the pregnancy and birth. You also have to get used to the needs of the baby. Both provide extra stress. Body image can also be a problem. Many new mothers feel fat. Mothers who breastfeed may lose extra pounds without much trouble. But it may still be six months or more before the old clothes fit.

Get Plenty of Rest—Don't Do Too Much

New mothers need to take it easy. They need to rest and to nap when the baby naps. If a new mother tries to do too much too soon, she can suddenly feel very tired. She may even faint. For the first few weeks after giving birth, plenty of rest is important. **New mothers who are well rested make better breastmilk. They also make more breastmilk than mothers who worry a lot or get too busy.**

Husband, family or friends can help with chores. Get someone else to help clean, shop for food, wash clothes, cook and care for older children during the first few weeks. New mothers do best when all they have to care for is themselves and the new baby. That's plenty!

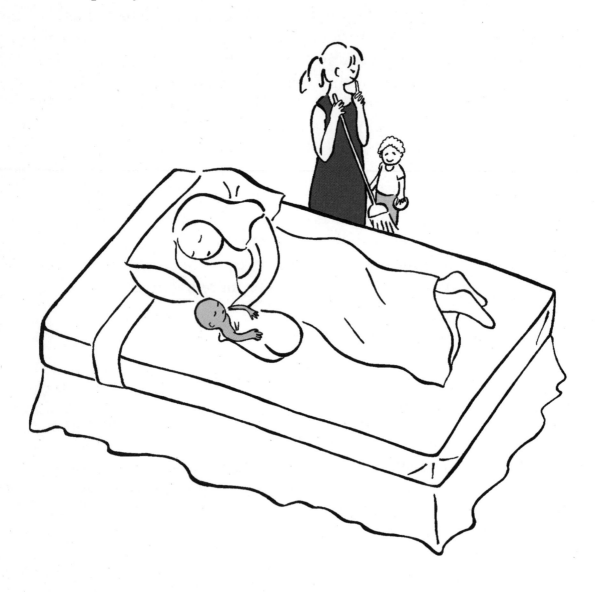

Bleeding

New mothers can expect vaginal bleeding for 2 to 6 weeks after childbirth. It's almost as if you'd "saved up" all those menstrual periods you missed. This is normal. The bleeding comes from the inside of the uterus where the placenta was attached. It continues until the healing in that area is complete.

Bleeding can be very heavy the first 3 to 5 days. Clots are not uncommon. Use hospital-size sanitary napkins. Old towels or pads can help protect your bed. The blood tends to "gush out" when you get up in the morning. Put something down on the floor beside the bed to prevent stains or spots on your carpet or floor.

The blood is bright-red for the first few days. Then it becomes watery. After that it will be dark-red, brown and even a bit yellow before it stops. It may also stop and start a few times before it's truly gone.

Sanitary napkins should be used to catch the blood, not tampons. Don't have sexual intercourse until the uterus is healed and the bleeding has stopped. Don't put anything into the vagina before healing is complete. It is easy for a new mother's uterus to become infected before it heals.

Mothers who breastfeed may have less bleeding. Breastfeeding makes the uterus contract. This helps heal the inside of the uterus. Eating plenty of dark-green vegetables and salads may speed healing and shorten the bleeding for some women. If you exercise too much in the first 6 weeks you may bleed longer. Too much exercise can also start the bleeding again if it had already stopped.

Trouble Signs

Call your doctor if you have any of these signs. They could mean trouble:

- **Extra-heavy bleeding,** which soaks through more than one large pad an hour, for several hours.

- **Bright-red bleeding** after the fourth day, especially if heavy.

- **Foul-smelling odor.** After-birth bleeding should smell like normal menstrual bleeding. A bad smell can be a sign of infection.

- **Abdominal cramping** that begins after the fourth day.

- **Extra-large clots.** Small clots, about half the size of a woman's thumb, are normal.

Showers Only, No Baths!

Don't take baths until after the bleeding stops. This cuts down the risk of infection. **Only showers or "sponge baths" should be taken.**

CAUTION: You may faint in the shower within the first week after giving birth. This is dangerous! A husband, family member or friend should stand by in the bathroom the first few times you shower. You might suddenly feel faint and need help.

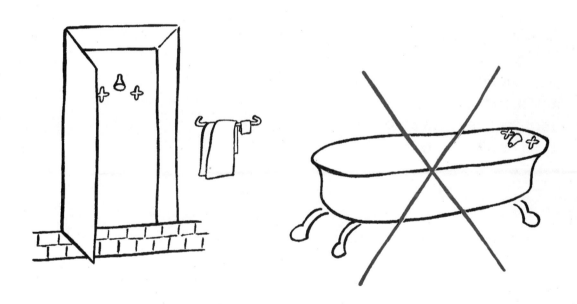

After-Birth Contractions

When you breastfeed a newborn, a hormone is released in your body that makes the uterus contract. This helps you get back into shape. Some of the same hormone is released when you see, hear, touch, hold or even *think* about your baby.

Most first-time mothers have little or no "after-birth contractions." Women who have had one or more children may feel strong abdominal cramping. These contractions come and go. They can feel as hurtful as the contractions of active labor. You may feel them for as long as 4 or 5 days.

Not every woman feels hurtful after-birth contractions. But if you do, relax and use slow, deep breathing. Be patient. After-birth contractions will pass. **Don't take aspirin** for the pain of after-birth contractions. Aspirin can lead to dangerous bleeding in new mothers. Stay away from other drugs, too. They go right into the breastmilk and to the baby.

Sore Bottom

The opening of your vagina may feel sore after you give birth. This soreness can last a few days whether or not you had stitches. There may also be some swelling. A cold pack can feel great. Make cold packs by soaking a large sanitary napkin in water. Squeeze out the extra water, and freeze it. You can make a dozen or more at a time. Whenever the coldness wears off, a new cold pack will be ready.

Care of Stitches

If you had stitches to repair a tear or a cut in your vaginal opening, be careful to keep the area clean. This helps to prevent infection and promotes quick healing. Wash the stitched area with a disinfectant (like Betadine®) after every visit to the toilet. Always wash from front to back. This may sting. But it helps prevent painful infections. You can also use antiseptic powder on the area after you have washed with the disinfectant.

Fluids

After giving birth, drink plenty of fluids. Drink at least 8 to 10 large glasses of water each day. This helps to replace fluids lost in childbirth. It also helps you make enough breastmilk.

Constipation

If you don't drink enough fluids your stools can become rock-hard and dry. You want to keep your stools soft and regular after giving birth. Hard stools are more difficult to pass. And if you strain you can get hemorrhoids.

These foods help keep your stools soft and regular. Eat plenty of them in the first few weeks after you give birth.

- fruits (fresh)
- dried fruits (like apricots and prunes)
- salads
- other vegetables
- 8-10 glasses of water each day
- whole grains
- prune juice
- flax seed
- beans

Extra Sweating

You may sweat a lot, even while you sleep. You may even drench your sheets and bed clothes. Heavy sweating is nature's way of getting rid of the extra fluids you needed during pregnancy. You no longer need extra blood and amniotic fluid. Once your normal fluid balance is back, the heavy sweating ends.

Fever

It is rare, but you may get a fever after giving birth. **Any fever that occurs in a woman within the first 2 weeks after childbirth can be dangerous. If you get a fever, call your doctor right away.**

Some women get a **low fever** when their milk "comes in." This passes in a day or two when the baby gets used to nursing. This *low* fever doesn't last long. It is nothing to worry about.

The Best Food for Babies

Breastmilk is a complete food. Baby doctors prefer mothers to breastfeed. Breastmilk provides **better nutrition than formulas.** Breastmilk is also **cheaper and easier** than formulas. It costs nothing. And it's **always fresh and ready.**

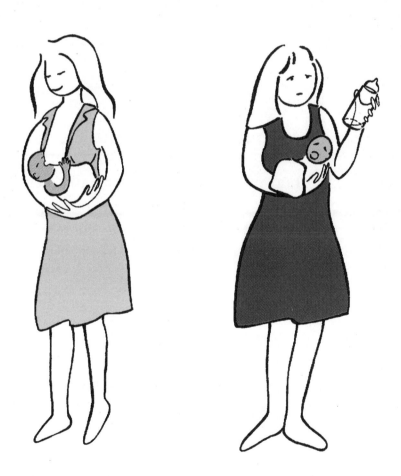

Protect Your Baby from Disease

Through your breastmilk, your baby can share in the immunity to disease you have built up over your lifetime. **Breastfed babies get fewer illnesses** than bottle-fed babies. And the illnesses they do get are often less severe.

Throughout the world doctors promote breastfeeding for healthier babies. Breastfeed your baby **at least through the first year of life.** Add soft foods and finger-foods between the 5th and the 8th month. Don't start these foods any sooner. And keep on breastfeeding, too! You know your child is ready for soft foods when he or she puts everything within reach into his or her mouth!

Protect Your Baby from Allergies

Breastfeeding is a good way to **reduce your baby's chance of getting allergies later in life**. Babies are never allergic to their own mother's milk. Sometimes a baby may react to breastmilk because of something the mother ate. The answer is to remove that food from your diet.

Babies **can** develop allergies when other foods, such as cow's milk, are started too soon. Cow's milk is the perfect food for a **calf.** But don't feed it to your baby during the first 12 months of life. **Feeding a baby cow's milk or formula with cow's milk in it can sometimes lead to a lifetime of allergies.**

Easy to Digest

Breastmilk is so easy to digest that a breastfed baby's stools have **no foul odor.** They are quite loose and shapeless. They range in color from yellow or mustard to green. And they have only a mild smell, which is not bad at all.

Formulas are harder for a baby to digest. Part of the formula can spoil inside the baby's intestines. This produces the strong, bad-smelling odor common to the stools of most bottle-fed babies. This also helps make gas, which can cause painful pressures and a crying, "colicky" baby. The stools of a baby on formula are also more solid. This makes them harder for the baby to push out.

Helps You Get Back into Shape

Breastfeeding helps you get back into shape in two ways. First, nursing your baby causes your body to release a hormone that helps contract or "shrink" your large uterus. **Breastfeeding helps pull your insides back into shape every time you nurse your baby.**

Second, when you nurse you make many quarts of milk each week. **Making milk burns up lots of calories.** This can help you to lose extra pounds after giving birth.

Helps Keep You Calm

Your body releases another hormone when you breastfeed. This one helps you feel patient, calm and relaxed when you nurse.

A Special Time

Mothers who breastfeed enjoy a special closeness with their babies. This can be a very special time. Besides the other good points, **breastfeeding can be a lot of fun!**

To Learn More about Breastfeeding

Books
> **Breastfeeding Your Baby**, by Jane Moody, Jane Britten and Karen Hogg (Fisher Books, 1997).

> **The Womanly Art of Breastfeeding, Revised Fifth Edition**, by La Leche League International (Plume, 1991).

You can also contact a La Leche League group. "La Leche" is Spanish and means "the milk." La Leche League is a nonprofit organization formed in 1956 by seven mothers. It provides free information and support to mothers who choose to breastfeed their babies. La Leche League has become highly respected worldwide. It now has more than 3,000 groups in 44 countries.

To find the La Leche League group nearest you, call your local library, the maternity department of your largest hospital, an obstetrician or pediatrician. Or you can contact La Leche League International. If you send them a self-addressed, stamped envelope, they will send you a list of the La Leche League groups and leaders nearest you at no charge. Contact: **La Leche League International, 1400 N. Meacham Rd., Schaumburg, IL 60173-4840.** You can call La Leche League toll-free at **1-800-LA-LECHE.** They can also be reached at **1-847-519-7730.**

CHILDBIRTH CLASSES

Being pregnant, giving birth and learning how to be a good parent—what adventures these are! Few things we do are as important or mean so much to us. Yet *most* of us are not very well prepared for *any* of these jobs.

If you are expecting a child, search out good childbirth classes. They are a fun way to prepare your body and your mind for the birth of your child. And they can help your birth be a much better experience. Women and men who attend childbirth classes tend to enjoy the birth process more than those who do not.

When you attend childbirth classes you can also learn how to reduce the risks and problems of pregnancy and birth for *both mother and child.*

A GUIDE TO HEALTHY EATING

(1) **Eat a wide variety of foods.** This will help ensure that the baby gets all the necessary ingredients for a strong, well-formed body.

(2) **Don't eat added sugars.** Cut out table sugar, syrups and sweets. If sugar or syrup is one of the first four ingredients listed on a package, *don't buy it!* These refined sugars give you empty calories. They can make you feel full. But they don't provide good nutrition for the baby. And they can help you gain too much weight.

(3) **Don't eat fatty or fried foods.** These are hard to digest. They can give you heartburn or indigestion. Pork and lamb take longer to digest than other meats. Eat less pork and lamb. Or don't eat them at all when you are pregnant.

(4) **Eat whole grains only.** This includes breads, cereals, rice, pastas and tortillas. When these products are made with the complete, whole grain they provide more food value for the baby. They are also full of fiber to help prevent constipation. Learn to read the labels on packages before you buy your food. Some breads made with white, refined grains contain food coloring. This makes them look like whole-grain bread. Don't buy bread if it has food coloring or dye in it. Real whole-grain bread will have no coloring added.

(5) **Eat smaller meals more often.** Women who skip meals during pregnancy can faint. This is dangerous for both mother and child.

When you are pregnant, your stomach and intestines get shoved and squished up and back by the growing uterus and baby. You no longer have room to handle a large meal. You will feel better if you eat smaller meals more often. Your meals will digest more easily.

Nausea is a common complaint of pregnancy. You can often prevent nausea by nibbling or "grazing" throughout the day. Morning sickness is nausea in the morning. You can sometimes prevent it if you eat a little snack right before going to bed or in the middle of the night. Or eat a little something, like crackers, before getting up in the morning.

(6) **Drink plenty of fluids,** especially water and juices. Many doctors ask pregnant women to drink at least **eight glasses of water each day.** You need more fluids when you are pregnant. Extra fluid helps support the increase in your blood volume. It also helps you maintain the amniotic fluid around the baby. Drinking more fluid can help you prevent constipation. Stay away from drinks that contain caffeine, like coffees, teas or colas. Don't drink anything that contains alcohol, either. Alcohol and caffeine can both cause problems during pregnancy.

24-Hour Diet Recall

__What to do__: Write down *everything* you ate in the last 24 hours.

Breakfast:

Snack:

Lunch:

Snack:

Dinner:

Snack:

Now, using the foods you have listed on this page, **fill in one day of the Diet Chart on the next page**. This will help you see how well you are eating for pregnancy. You will also learn what foods you may not be eating enough of.

Diet Worksheet

(Week Starting _____)

FOOD GROUP	SUNDAY					MONDAY					TUESDAY					WEDNESDAY				
	Daily Servings					Daily Servings					Daily Servings					Daily Servings				
	1	2	3	4	5	1	2	3	4	5	1	2	3	4	5	1	2	3	4	5
Protein Foods	❑	❑	❑	❑		❑	❑	❑	❑		❑	❑	❑	❑		❑	❑	❑	❑	
Milk & Milk Prod.	❑	❑	❑	❑+❑*		❑	❑	❑	❑+❑*		❑	❑	❑	❑+❑*		❑	❑	❑	❑+❑*	
Breads & Cereals	❑	❑	❑	❑		❑	❑	❑	❑		❑	❑	❑	❑		❑	❑	❑	❑	
Vitamin C Fruits & Vegs	❑					❑					❑					❑				
Fruits & Vegs: dark green leafy & yellow	❑	❑				❑	❑				❑	❑				❑	❑			
Other Fruits & Vegs	❑	❑				❑	❑				❑	❑				❑	❑			

FOOD GROUP	THURSDAY					FRIDAY					SATURDAY				
	Daily Servings					Daily Servings					Daily Servings				
	1	2	3	4	5	1	2	3	4	5	1	2	3	4	5
Protein Foods	❑	❑	❑	❑		❑	❑	❑	❑		❑	❑	❑	❑	
Milk & Milk Prod.	❑	❑	❑	❑+❑*		❑	❑	❑	❑+❑*		❑	❑	❑	❑+❑*	
Breads & Cereals	❑	❑	❑	❑		❑	❑	❑	❑		❑	❑	❑	❑	
Vitamin C Fruits & Vegs	❑					❑					❑				
Fruits & Vegs: dark green leafy & yellow	❑	❑				❑	❑				❑	❑			
Other Fruits & Vegs	❑	❑				❑	❑				❑	❑			

Check off for the week: Liver (1 serving) ❑
* For Pregnant Teenagers or Breastfeeding Moms

Make copies of this page to keep track of your diet.

FOOD GROUPS AND SERVINGS

Protein Servings:
- Meat (2 ounces)
- Eggs (2)
- Seeds or nuts (1/2 cup)
- Fish (2 ounces)
- Beans (3/4 cup)
- Nut butter (1/4 cup or 4 tablespoons)

A quarter-pound hamburger would be 2 protein servings. A chicken drumstick would be 1 serving. A chicken thigh would also be 1 serving. But half a chicken breast would be 2 servings. (Nuts and seeds are high in fat.)

Milk and Milk Products:
- Milk (1 cup)
- Cottage cheese (1-1/3 cups)
- Kefir (1 cup)
- Ice cream (1-1/2 cups)
- Yogurt (1 cup)
- Cheese (1-1/2 slices or a 1-1/2-inch cube)

Any kind of milk will do. Whole milk, nonfat, 2%, 1%, powdered or buttermilk are all fine. (Ice cream is high in fat.)

Bread and Cereals:
- Bread (1 slice)
- Grains, such as rice, bulgur, oats, couscous (1/2 cup)
- Pasta (1/2 cup)
- Bagel (1/2)
- English muffin (1/2)
- Buns and rolls (about 1 per serving)
- Tortillas (3 corn tortillas make 2 servings; 1 flour tortilla makes 2 servings)
- Cooked cereal, such as oatmeal or cream of wheat (1/2 cup)
- Dry cereal, such as corn flakes or raisin bran (3/4 cup)

Vitamin-C Fruits and Vegetables:
- Tomatoes (1 medium)
- Grapefruit (1 medium)
- Pineapple (3/4 cup)
- Oranges (1 medium)
- Lemon (1 medium)
- Strawberries (3/4 cup)

Eat these fruits fresh and raw if you can. Heat destroys vitamin C in fruits or fruit juice. So does exposure to air.

Dark-green Leafy or Yellow Fruits and Vegetables:
(1 serving is 1 cup raw or 3/4 cup cooked)

- Romaine lettuce
- Chard
- Bok choy
- Asparagus
- Spinach
- Kale
- Brussels sprouts

These are some of the *dark*-green vegetables. Eat at least half of your greens each week raw, in salads. (Iceberg lettuce is *not* dark green!)

- Apricots
- Peaches
- Mangoes
- Sweet potatoes
- Yellow and orange squash
- Nectarines
- Papayas
- Yams
- Carrots
- Pumpkin

These are some dark-yellow (or orange) vegetables and fruits. One serving is also 1 cup raw or 3/4 cup cooked.

Other Fruits and Vegetables:
(1 serving is 1 cup raw or 3/4 cup cooked)

- Apples
- Plums
- Figs
- Beets
- Corn
- Pears
- Bananas
- Potatoes
- Turnips
- Green beans
- Peas
- Squash (not yellow or orange), such as zucchini

Note: These dietary recommendations have been adapted by Christine L. Vega, M.P.H., R.D., from the State of California Department of Health W.I.C. program guidelines (Women, Infants and Children supplemental feeding program).

INDEX

sign of first stage of labor, 74
nature of, in first-stage labor, 76, 78
painful. *See* transition, signs of
pushing (second-stage labor), 71
third-stage labor, 92
after childbirth, 108
cramping, 53
crowning, 88

D
diabetes of pregnancy, 68
diaphragm, 42-45
diet, 35, 38, 56-59, 116-121
dilation. *See* cervix, first-stage labor
   (dilation)
drugs, 61, 62
   prescription, 63
drugs while breastfeeding, 108

E
edema, 54, 66
effacing. *See* cervix, thinning of
egg, 22-27
embryo, 26, 28
exercise, 51, 57
   aerobic, 53

F
fainting, 107
Fallopian tubes, 22-26
fats, 58, 116, 120
fertilization. *See* conception
fetus, 28-33
fever, 110

H
heart, 42, 43, 45
heartburn. *See* indigestion
hemorrhoids, 53
heroin, 63
hiccuping. *See* transition, signs of
hot flashes. *See* transition, signs of

I
incontinence, 49
indigestion, 116, 117
intestines, 42-45
implantation, 26
irritability. *See* transition, signs of

J
jaundice, 102
jogging, 53
junk foods, 57, 59

K
Kegel, Dr. Arnold, 48
kegel muscle, 48-51
kicking (by the baby), 30

L
La Leche League, 114
labor, first-stage
   definition, 69-71
   easier, 57
   false, 73, 74
   length of, 77
   signs of, 72-75
   slowing of, 54
labor, second-stage, 82, 85-90
labor, third-stage, 91, 92
liver, 42-45

M
medication, 62, 63
menstrual blood, 24, 26
menstruation, 21, 24
morning sickness. *See* nausea
mother, the first week
   the blues, 103
   diet, 109
   excessive perspiration, 110
   need for rest, 103, 104
   stresses, 103, 104
mucous plug
   definition, 41
   loss of, 72-74

V

W

Notes

Notes